Cracking the Menopause Code

A Candid Guide for the Perimenopausal and Menopausal Woman to Blossom During the Change

Bernice Pond

CRACKING THE MENOPAUSE CODE

© Copyright 2019 Bernice POND - All rights reserved.

The content contained within this book may not be reproduced, duplicated or transmitted without direct written permission from the author or the publisher.

Under no circumstances will any blame or legal responsibility be held against the publisher, or author, for any damages, reparation, or monetary loss due to the information contained within this book. Either directly or indirectly.

Legal Notice:

This book is copyright protected. This book is only for personal use. You cannot amend, distribute, sell, use, quote or paraphrase any part, or the content within this book, without the consent of the author or publisher.

Disclaimer Notice:

Please note the information contained within this document is for educational and entertainment purposes only. All effort has been executed to present accurate, up to date, and reliable, complete information. No warranties of any kind are declared or implied. Readers acknowledge that the author is not engaging in the rendering of legal, financial, medical or professional advice. The content within this book has been derived from various sources. Please consult a licensed professional before attempting any techniques outlined in this book.

By reading this document, the reader agrees that under no circumstances is the author responsible for any losses, direct or indirect, which are incurred as a result of the use of the information contained within this document, including, but not limited to, — errors, omissions, or inaccuracies.

CRACKING THE MENOPAUSE CODE

TABLE OF CONTENTS

1. Introduction — Pg 8

2. How Do You Know If You Are Premenopausal — Pg 14

3. What Is the Menopause? — Pg 37

4. Managing the Menopause? — Pg 58

5. What Happens to My Brain During the Menopause? — Pg 80

6. What are the Pros and Cons of HRT? — Pg 101

7. What are the Pros and Cons of Using Natural Alternatives to HRT? — Pg 117

8. How to Look After your Mental Health and Wellbeing During the Menopause — Pg 129

9. Maintaining Good Relations at Home and Work — Pg 154

10. Staying Fit and Healthy During the Menopause — Pg 169

| 11 | Final Words | Pg 189 |
| 12 | Bibliography | Pg 196 |

Introduction

It's your time of the month, and your period has not arrived. The only other time this happened to you was during pregnancy. Could you be pregnant? No, that would be impossible. You wait a few more days, but still no period. You begin to worry. Could this be the first symptom of reproductive cancer? Finally, your period starts, but it is very heavy. This worries you even more.

You make an appointment with your gynaecologist. When you finally get to see your doctor, she has some information for you that is quite shocking – you have entered the perimenopause. What is that? Is it the same as the menopause? Your heart sinks as you feel older than your age. Unable to ask your doctor any questions to relieve your anxiety, you go home to be alone with your thoughts. The doctor said it was a natural process, and there wasn't anything you must do to treat it. Still, you have so many questions, but whom can you ask?

In generations past, women had their mother and aunts to model going through the menopause. However, time and distance are separating you from family and the knowledge they could pass on to you. Conversely, you are too shy to ask your friends. the menopause, or the change, seems to be a very sensitive subject as it never enters social conversations. Hoping to find answers, you go online and purchase a couple of e-books, but neither book makes any sense to you.

My name is Bernice Pond. I'm here to answer all your burning questions (no pun intended) with compassion and care. I hope to share the knowledge I have gleaned from my forty-year career as a registered nurse in the United Kingdom. During my many years as a nurse, I have witnessed many women go through the change. I have also taken the journey from menstruation to the menopause and witnessed my friends and colleagues make the same journey. One day my daughter will also embark down this path, and I don't want her to make this journey alone. I want to give her some sound knowledge of what the menopause is all about.

I lost my mother before I could ask her any

questions about the menopause. Losing my mother was naturally a painful experience. I have written this book for my daughter, and women like you, who are seeking advice and guidance. In this book, I will enable and empower you to understand the physical and emotional changes you will go through. I will also help you to navigate through the rollercoaster ride that is known as "the change."

I was fifty-one years old when I discovered that the menopause had become a reality for me. Over the years, I have nursed patients through the most challenging parts of their lives. I know from personal experience what a challenge it is to make the natural journey through the menopause.

With my help and expertise, you will be fully armed with all the information you need to unravel the myths surrounding the natural processes that every woman goes through. After reading my book, *Cracking The Menopause Code*, you will be able to talk to friends and colleagues about the menopause with confidence. Each chapter in this book will provide you with actionable steps. The book will help you to understand the symptoms, issues, and complications of the menopause. Besides, the book will offer practical information regarding hormone replacement therapy (HRT), natural alternatives, and how to keep yourself fit and healthy the natural and safe way.

There are many ways to go through the menopause. Some women sail through it with a sense of denial. Others experience every symptom that there is, but they suffer in silence. However, this is not the way to successfully navigate the menopause. You don't have to be without the information needed to make your journey through the menopause easy and unflustered.

As with any medical issue, many research studies contradict themselves. The media grabs onto sensational facts that give birth to confusion and panic. Even some doctors do not agree on how to treat women that are going through the menopause. There are studies in favour of HRT and studies against it. Whom can you believe? Do you find yourself relating to the following situations?

1. There is no one to ask about the menopause.

2. The people you seek support from do not have any useful information.

3. There are countless myths surrounding the menopause; you can't separate fact from fiction.

4. There is such a shroud of mystery around the menopause; you feel clueless.

5. That the menopause is such a taboo subject that you can't talk about it in a social situation.

If you follow this guide, you will be able to understand what is happening to your mind and body. You will also be able to understand the various stages of the menopause and gain a positive outlook on a natural part of your life. After reading this book, you will be able to talk to your doctor with confidence and calmly assess the right path to take for your unique journey through the menopause.

My book is meant to help you navigate through "the change." I understand that many myths have worked themselves into our modern psyche. Some of them are:

- The only symptom you suffer from during the menopause is hot flushes.

- Your period will suddenly stop one day.
- Everyone experiences hot flushes the same way.
- There is no treatment or cure for hot flushes.
- HRT is dangerous and can cause cancer.
- After the menopause, you will no longer have a sex drive.
- The menopause causes weight gain.
- The menopause causes an overactive bladder.
- The menopause is a terrible ordeal.

Let us battle myth with facts. In this, I will give you the benefit of my experience as a nursing health professional, alongside the latest research. Are you ready to shine a light on a subject that has been shrouded in myth and mystery? Are you ready to blossom during the change? Good. I want to thank you in advance for letting me into your confidence. Let us begin our journey together…

Chapter One: How Do You Know If You Are Premenopausal?

As women, we go through many phases of life. We start our menstruation when we move to adulthood, where we have the choice of whether to have children. Then, the years pass, and we arrive at the perimenopause. It is here that we begin the fantastic journey that is the menopause. The menopause does not happen without warning. It sends its friend the perimenopause to say hello. The signs and symptoms of the perimenopause differ for each woman. Some women do not even realise they are in the perimenopausal state.

What is the Perimenopause?

The perimenopause (or the premenopausal stage) is the state before reaching the menopause. The perimenopause is not severe or painful. Many women go into this state as early as their mid-thirties, but usually, the change begins in your forties. A common sign that you are in the perimenopause might be the irregularity of your periods. Specifically, your period stops some months but begin again without warning. Also, the flow of your period may change from heavy to light or from light to heavy.

The Symptoms of the Perimenopause

The symptoms of the perimenopause are very similar to the menopause except for the irregular periods. When you are in the menopause your periods stop altogether. During the perimenopause, your body may stop ovulating or releasing an egg every month. However, you still might be releasing eggs, so you want to keep taking measures not to get pregnant.

When we are born, we have a certain amount of eggs stored inside of us. No one knows the exact count or the month we will run out of eggs. At an early age, we begin menstruation, and slowly every month, we shed the lining of our uterus if the egg does not get fertilised. When you start the perimenopause, your periods become irregular. Ovulation no longer runs like clockwork, and there will be months that we do not release an egg and start our period. There will be times when the days between periods are either cut short or increased. The number of days between periods can be a sign as to whether you are in early or late perimenopause. As a rule, if your period comes more than seven days late, you are in early perimenopause. However, if there is a more than a sixty-day gap between your periods, you are probably in late perimenopause.

When your oestrogen level decreases, you may begin to have symptoms caused by this decrease. It is common to have headaches, breast tenderness, weight gain, and hot flushes. Not all women experience the perimenopause in the same way. The perimenopause comes around eight to ten years ahead of the menopause, so you might not get all the signs at one time. Usually, you experience the perimenopause between the ages of thirty to forty years old.

As a woman gets older, changes start to happen that trigger the reproductive systems to behave differently than when a woman is young. Just as our hormones started our periods, our hormones will start the perimenopause with a drop-in oestrogen, produced by the ovaries. In fact, during our cycle of menstruation, oestrogen levels will go up and down during our twenty-eight day-cycle. The fluctuation in oestrogen levels is what sets off irregular periods.

The Menstruation Cycle

First the follicle-stimulating hormone (FSH) stimulates the fluid-filled sacs in the ovaries (follicles) to produce oestrogen. When the oestrogen gets to a certain level, the brain tells your pituitary gland to turn off follicle-stimulating hormone (FSH) and create a surge of luteinising hormone (LH). This surge causes the ovary to release an egg from the follicle, and then we ovulate. The left-over follicle produces progesterone and oestrogen. If you don't get pregnant, your progesterone level goes down, and this signals the start of your period. As you can see, a delicate process occurs every month due to the hormones our body creates. When these processes become altered, change begins to occur. The perimenopause marks the first phase of bodily changes in a woman.

Oestrogen levels rising and dropping within our bodies trigger differences in our cycle. The ovaries are starting to shut down the production of oestrogen, and the perimenopause is triggered as a result. Eventually, the ovaries will produce such a low level of oestrogen, and you will no longer release an egg. When this happens, your period will stop, and then you will begin the journey into the menopause. If you have undergone surgery for a hysterectomy, it may trigger the perimenopause (if you have not yet gone through the menopause). Also, chemo or radiation can trigger the perimenopause.

The perimenopause is nature's way of easing you into the change, and there is no reason to stress about it. These are some of the key symptoms that are associated with the perimenopause:

- Irregular periods.
- Headaches.
- Loss of sex drive.

- Increase in heartbeat.
- Weight gain.
- Hair changes.
- Breast tenderness.
- Worse PMS before your period.
- Periods are either heavier or lighter than usual.

The perimenopause is the gentle start of the menopause. It's possible not to feel any significant symptoms. You might not notice anything out of the ordinary at first. You could start having bouts of insomnia or mood swings and think a stressful situation is causing them. You could even feel a bit depressed. However, once you start having night sweats, hot flushes, and frequent urination a warning bell might go off. There is nothing like a hot flush to signal that your body is going through changes.

Change in Your Body

By the time you approach your late thirties, you are not producing as much progesterone, and the number of quality follicles is diminishing. The body produces a lower level of the hormone oestrogen, and as a result, you are not ovulating as much. As you reach your forties, your level of oestrogen rises and falls, and the body produces more FSH to signal the ovaries to produce more oestrogen. With all these different hormone fluctuations, you will begin to have various symptoms. During your forties, you start to experience many significant events within your personal and working life. It also signals the beginning of mid-life events such as children leaving home and parents getting ill and dying. These mid-life events also affect your moods, making it hard to distinguish whether the perimenopause causes depression and irritability or not.

Pay Special Attention to These Symptoms

The key to the perimenopause is that you have not ceased your period. Your flow may be light or heavy, but your periods still present, albeit irregular. It's not necessary to visit the doctor when you reach the perimenopause stage, but there are some warning signs that may need your attention. They are the following:

- Spotting after your period.
- Blood clots during your period.
- Bleeding after sex.
- Your periods that are either shorter or longer than usual.

These irregularities could be a sign of fibroids, hormonal imbalances, and in extreme cases, cancer. You also have every right to call your doctor if one or more of the symptoms of the perimenopause interferes with your daily routine. You do not have to suffer in silence. There are things that you can do to alleviate the symptoms of the perimenopause.

When Your Body Burns Hotter Than the Sun

Hot flushes are the most common physiological change in women starting the perimenopause. No one knows precisely what causes a hot flush or why it occurs. They do know that oestrogen is involved but not precisely how a hot flush is triggered. It is the sudden feeling of heat that seems to burn throughout your whole body. You can stand in front of the freezer to feel more relaxed, but it feels like even if you were in the middle of Antarctica, you would still be burning up. The burning sensation may begin in your upper cheeks and spread throughout your body. You may feel an acute heat on your face. The reason you feel so hot is that the blood vessels near your skin's surface widen to cool off. This reaction makes you break out into a sweat. The medical name for hot flushes is vasomotor symptoms.

Between thirty-five and fifty per cent of all women will experience hot flushes or night sweats during their change. Hot flushes feel like having waves of heat passing through you. These hot flushes can happen in full force to some women, and in others, they will be a mild episode. It is the first sign that the perimenopause is starting. Two out of ten women will not have any hot flushes, and some women will only experience hot flushes for a limited time. Some women experience hot flushes for between seven to eleven years! If you are one of these women, don't panic; there are things you can do to ease or prevent them.

If you time a hot flush, you may find that it only lasts thirty seconds to a few minutes. The strange warm and burning feeling that you experience is not permanent; it will subside, and you can get on with your life. When they happen, explaining to your partner, companion, or children will help keep everyone calm and supportive. Before you turn to your doctor for help, there are some triggers that you can eliminate to decrease your hot flushes and make them less severe. Here are the most common triggers:

- Cigarette smoke.
- Stress.
- Heat.
- Tight clothing.
- Spicy foods.
- Caffeine.
- Alcohol.

It is possible to survive a hot flush; it just takes a little effort. You can create a pillow filled with water or buy a pillow that stays cool at night. You can wear looser fitting nightgowns that are lightweight and made from cotton. There are also breathing techniques that you can use to get through the hot flush — slow abdominal breathing taking in six to eight breaths per minute. Deep breathing for periods of fifteen minutes in the morning, noon, and evening can help to centre yourself and get you through the hot flushes.

Another great tip is to use daily exercise to calm your hot flushes. Try taking a soothing swim, going for a walk in the park or cycling through your local neighbourhood. There are natural supplements that you can take like black cohosh. Some doctors recommend eating food that is rich in soy like tofu or edamame to help lessen the periods of hot flushes. Your doctor may even feel that Hormone Replacement Therapy (HRT) is needed. We will discuss the pros and cons of Hormone Replacement Therapy in chapter five.

When you are experiencing a hot flush, you might notice that you become flushed. Your skin turns red, and you will also experience sweating as if you are in a sauna. Some women experience night sweats where they drench their sheets with perspiration. You may wake up and feel like someone threw a bucket of water on you. You might also feel anxious and observe that your heart is racing. Don't panic; this is all just part of the hot flush experience. Welcome to the club.

Other Events During the Perimenopause

Vaginal dryness is also something that a lowered level of oestrogen may bring about. It is caused as vaginal tissue starts to get thinner and drier, which also causes a loss of elasticity and natural lubrication. These changes can lead to pain and discomfort and cause your sex life to decline. The loss of oestrogen can also make you more susceptible to urinary and vaginal infections. Also, the loss of tone in your tissues may cause some urinary incontinence.

Uterine bleeding can occur when a lowered level of progesterone interferes with the regular rate of growth in the endometrium (lining of the uterus). The growth, a thicker lining in the uterus, results in more substantial periods. There may also be fibroids (benign tumours) and endometrial tissue found outside the uterine wall. These growths are fuelled and controlled by oestrogen. The lining of the uterus may be located outside of the uterus itself. Fibroids and endometrial tissue build-up can be a problem, that needs to be monitored and sometimes dealt with surgically.

Up to forty per cent of women going through the perimenopause complain about insomnia and sleep disturbances. Some perimenopausal women feel that having night sweats is the reason they cannot sleep. Sleep disturbances can be caused by different issues or events that occur within the body, so it's hard to determine if the cause is the perimenopause. Sometimes insomnia is a sign of ageing, as both men and women may experience trouble sleeping as they get older.

When it comes to mood changes, ten to twenty per cent of women have reported their moods have been affected by the perimenopause. However, at present, there has not been a hormonal link to mood changes such as irritability and depression. Doctors seem to think that ageing is the cause of these mood swings. However, the jury is still out. Another change that some women report is difficulty concentrating. Oestrogen and progesterone have a part in supporting brain function. However, there are no confirmed scientific or medical links between cognitive functions and the perimenopause.

What Does the Term 'Premature Menopause' Mean?

The early menopause is when you begin the perimenopause or the menopause at an early age. This is generally acknowledged as any woman under the age of forty-five who experiences menopausal symptoms. There are various reasons for this condition. Some of them are:

- Chromosome abnormalities, such as Turner Syndrome. Turner Syndrome occurs where a girl is born with only one normal X sex chromosome (we usually have two). The girl will have underdeveloped ovaries as a result of this chromosomal abnormality.

- Autoimmune disease - the immune system targets and attacks body tissues.
- Infections such as mumps, malaria and tuberculosis (very rare).
- Cancer treatments, such as radiotherapy and chemotherapy.
- Removal of the ovaries due to a hysterectomy.
- POI (Primary Ovarian insufficiency).

What is Primary Ovarian Insufficiency (POI)?

Primary ovarian insufficiency (POI) happens when women under forty have very few periods and elevated follicle-stimulating hormone (FSH) levels. This may be a sign that the woman has fewer eggs in her ovaries. In ninety per cent of cases of primary ovarian insufficiency, the root cause is still unknown. Research has determined that the follicles, small sacs in the ovaries, are not working well. Further, there are fewer working follicles than usual. The cause of the follicle problems is still unknown. The symptoms of primary ovarian insufficiency are like those of the perimenopause.

Individuals suffer from hot flushes, night sweats, irritability, poor concentration, decreased sex drive, and vaginal dryness. The difference is mostly that these symptoms are caused by something going wrong – not the natural result of the menopause. If you are under the age of forty-five and have any of these symptoms, seek medical attention.

Surgical Menopause

The surgical menopause is triggered when a hysterectomy and removal of the ovaries take place. Having a hysterectomy is a highly stressful and life-changing event. To illustrate the realities of the surgical menopause upon a young lady, a dear friend has kindly agreed to share her story. The following is Anne's story, in her own words.

The night before Christmas, Anne felt a sudden and sharp pain in her back. The pain was as intense as a contraction, but it didn't build and then finish like a contraction. It was just one very intense and sharp pain. Along with the pain, Anne had nausea and eventually threw up. She had no idea what was going on. She also noticed that she had spotted her underwear as if she was starting a period. Unable to take the pain, Anne went to the emergency room where she was told that it was probably a kidney stone. There was urine in her blood and the pain was in the area that a kidney stone would be. The nurse practitioner ordered a CT scan and managed Anne's pain with morphine.

An hour later, after the results of the CT scan were in, the nurse informed Anne that she had a mass near her ovary and not kidney stones. An ultrasound was ordered to determine if the ovary was twisted. If this happened, she would need to immediately undergo surgery. After the ultrasound, the nurse practitioner informed Anne that the ovary was not twisted, and she could go home. Anne was referred to a gynaecologist for further treatment and released. The sharp pain went away, and Anne was able to resume her usual routine.

A month after waiting for an appointment, Anne saw a gynaecologist who had been sent the CT scan and ultrasound. She informed Anne that the mass was a cyst and urgent surgery was required. There was also a higher risk of ovarian cancer due to Anne's family history, her obesity and pre-diabetes. Consequently, the gynaecologist told Anne that a hysterectomy was needed. Anne had read about surgical menopause and asked the gynaecologist if this would happen to her. The gynaecologist asked her when she had noticed her last period. Anne said a year ago but that she had been spotting. The gynaecologist said that based on her age and the absence of menstruation, Anne had probably gone through the menopause already and would not be affected by the removal of her uterus, fallopian tubes, ovaries and cervix.

When the day arrived, Anne prepared for the operation and had some sad feelings about the hysterectomy. Due to complications, Anne needed to undergo a second operation. The second surgery went well, the cyst was removed, and a hysterectomy had been performed. Anne went home after a night in the hospital where the doctor had ordered pain management. The surgery had been done robotically, so Anne only had four small incisions on her abdomen. The pain was minimal.

In the weeks that followed, Anne saw a therapist and talked about the loss of her reproductive organs. She was also feeling very emotional and fatigued from the surgery and suffered hot flushes and night sweats. The operation had "awakened" her menopause symptoms, and she experienced surgical menopause. Anne recovered quickly from the surgery and came to terms with her loss. After a few weeks, the menopause symptoms disappeared, and she was back to being herself.

Does the Perimenopause Affect Your Mental Health?

Medically, there has not been a link between depression and the perimenopause; however, many women experience an emotional surge when the "change" happens. It stands to reason that when we reach the end of an era, we get sentimental. After having a period for almost forty years, you approach the end of something that has been with you for a long time. You will no longer have to shop for feminine health products or worry about your period starting at an unexpected moment. Besides, your relationship with the obstetrician and gynaecologist will change. Once you visited your obstetrician or gynaecologist monthly to check on your pregnancy; you are now seeing them at the end of an era. It is good that we have the perimenopause to help us with the transition into not being able to conceive anymore.

Perhaps you did not have children. If that is something you feel is lacking in your life, the perimenopause can be very emotional. You might even think that you must rush out and try to get pregnant before the "end" comes. Alternatively, you feel good about the fact that you did not have children, but still, it makes you pause and realise that a new cycle of life is starting. The perimenopause is the chance to ease into the change of the menopause. The key to the perimenopause is that the symptoms come and go. Where there is a month that you have hot flushes, there can be a month or several months that you don't have them — the same with your periods. You can still ovulate and get pregnant. However, please be aware that during the perimenopause, you may not be releasing an ovum.

In this stage of your life, you are going through

many changes. Your children are growing up and needing you less. Alternatively, maybe you have conquered empty nest syndrome, but you find that your parents need you to help them through their ageing process. You might be retiring from a job that you have held for many years. Consequently, your day-to-day life is changing, and you must adapt to it. Then comes the perimenopause and your body is signalling that a tremendous change is beginning to happen. The perimenopause is the start of a substantial change in your body. If you feel that you are in the perimenopause, you do not need to stress. Pay attention to your symptoms and remember that it is reasonable to seek medical attention if the symptoms are so pronounced, they are interfering with your daily routine. Only your doctor can tell you for sure if you are in a perimenopausal state. We, as women, are lucky to have the stage of the perimenopause to prepare for significant change.

Chapter Summary

The perimenopause happens before the menopause and has symptoms that are very much like the menopause. During the perimenopause, fluctuations in oestrogen levels affect your menstrual cycle. Some women cease having a regular menstrual cycle during the perimenopause. A woman's emotions may be influenced by either the surge of hormones or the decrease in hormones. If any symptoms of the perimenopause affect your daily routine, you may want to seek medical help. In the next chapter, we will delve further into the meaning and symptoms of the menopause.

Chapter Two: What Is the Menopause?

As we move deeper into the ageing process, our body changes in many ways. We start to see grey in our hair. We begin to gain a bit of weight around our hips, bums and tums. The things we once did with ease in the past become harder to do. Still, we are active and vital. Our bodies are fit and healthy, and our minds are full of beautiful memories and hopes for the future. We have struggled to change unhealthy habits, and we have added new habits to make our life easier. If our minds have changed over the years, what about our bodies? Is there any change? After years of planning our lives around the menstrual cycle, we are finally getting to the end of an era. Our periods are about to disappear forever. This change may startle you or make you jump with joy. Whatever the reaction, it is essential to understand what is or what has happened to you.

Counting the Months

If you are over forty years old, you may have already been experiencing irregular periods. You may have gone months without a period, only to have a heavy or very light period when it finally arrives. It is important to note because, after each cycle, you should begin to count how many months you have not menstruated. For example, your last period was in January, but you have no period during February and March. So, begin your count from February. It takes a full year of going without your periods to determine whether you are going through the menopause or not. For example, if your menopause date starts in February, but then you have another period in April, you must start counting all over again. Finally, you have not had any periods for a year – you know you are now in the midst of the menopause. Before you are diagnosed as being in the menopause, you have probably gone through the perimenopause. We discussed the perimenopause in the last chapter.

How to Tell the Difference Between the Perimenopause and the Menopause

If the symptoms are so similar, how do you know which stage you have reached? Well, the main symptom is that you have not had a period in a year. The other symptoms, like hot flushes and night sweats, you may have already experienced. Does this mean that you will have more symptoms now that you are in the menopause? We will examine the answers these questions within this chapter.

Sometimes it is hard to understand that although you experience the same type of symptoms during the perimenopause as you do in the menopause, they are two different stages. The most crucial difference between the perimenopause and the menopause is that your periods have stopped. The postmenopause occurs after you stop menstruating altogether. The good news is that as you move forward in time, some of the symptoms of the menopause stop on their own. You will not be plagued with hot flushes for the rest of your life. Your body begins to adjust. If you get your period after a long time of not menstruating, it might be time to go to your doctor, especially if the flow is not like your regular flow. Certain gynaecological conditions may be causing you to bleed unrelated to your period. Also, see your doctor if you experience sharp pains or unfamiliar pains that accompany the bleeding.

For most of your life, the ovaries have been in control of your menstruation cycle. As they decline and stop working, you go through many bodily changes. The most crucial difference is that your period stops happening each month. The ovaries are shutting down and not producing enough oestrogen and progesterone. Primarily this happens in your early fifties. The shutdown can also occur if you have had an illness such as cancer, that needed to be treated with radiation or chemotherapy. Another reason the shutdown can happen is if you had a hysterectomy and your ovaries were taken out along with your uterus, cervix, and fallopian tubes.

How Will I Be Diagnosed with the Menopause?

To diagnose the menopause, your doctor or

physician will ask you the date of your last menstrual cycle. These dates are important for your doctor to determine if you have reached the menopause. For a woman under fifty years old, a physician will be looking at a two-year absence of menstruation. For a woman over fifty years old, a physician will be looking at a year-long lack of menstruation. Usually, a doctor will use the cessation of menstruation and history of menopausal symptoms to determine if you are in the menopause. There is typically no urine or blood testing done.

The general rule of thumb in deciding whether to seek medical attention is if the symptom interferes with your lifestyle. For example, some women might only experience hot flushes in certain situations like drinking alcohol. They will not suffer a hot flush at any other time. If you find that hot flushes are keeping you from doing routine activities such as sleeping or going to work, you may want to see a doctor or physician. They can help in either prescribing you medication or helping you to understand other options for dealing with the full-blown symptoms of the menopause. Unfortunately, there is no one size fits all treatment for the menopause. It's best to speak to a physician and talk to them about your symptoms. They can help you to rule out any illness not related to the menopause. Also, your gynaecologist will be familiar with your medical history and be able to prescribe the best source of treatment for you.

What Are Hormones, and How Do They Affect the Onset of the Menopause?

Hormones are the messengers that transport messages to all areas of our body. Hormones affect the physical and chemical systems of our body. These hormones can shut processes down, start them up, speed them up or slow them down. Oestrogen and progesterone are mainly found in a woman's reproductive system and are responsible for both your fertility and menstruation. Two other hormones support the reproductive system. These hormones are known as luteinizing hormone (LH) and follicle-stimulating hormone (FSH). These hormones come into play during your menstrual cycle. However, when you enter the menopause, these hormones no longer perform their functions as regulators of oestrogen, progesterone, and testosterone. This happens because the amount of oestrogen has lessened to the point that the ovarian follicles and ovaries become less responsive.

As you move from the perimenopause and into the menopause, your ovaries begin to produce progressively less of the vital hormone known as oestrogen. When you get to the menopause; the ovaries are producing very little oestrogen. When this happens, your breasts become tender, and you feel bloated. You also may have headaches, night sweats, hot flushes, insomnia, vaginal dryness, fatigue, and bone loss. These are just some of the symptoms that may occur at this sensitive time.

Oestrogen plays a big part in our reproductive system. Oestrogen is the star because it keeps our female reproductive organs in good shape. Here is a list of the incredible things that oestrogen does for our body:

- It regulates vaginal elasticity and moisture.
- It allows the healthy blood flow to the vagina.

- It is responsible for thickening the uterus lining during the menstrual cycle.
- It assists with the health and preservation of our bones and skeletal structure.
- It oversees sexual development in your body and your menstrual cycle

There are three significant types of oestrogen: Estrone, Estradiol and Estriol. In general, oestrogen handles many processes in a woman's body. I have discussed how oestrogen promotes menstruation, but it is also responsible for our sexual behaviour, mainly our sex drive. When we have a decrease in oestrogen, our sex drive is affected. Oestrogen is also responsible for the maturing and preservation of the vagina and uterus. This crucial hormone is also in charge of ovarian functions, such as the development of ovarian follicles.

Estrone (E1) is produced from the sex hormone androgen. A biochemical process called aromatisation changes androgen into estrone. Throughout the menopause, estrone is the only oestrogen produced by the ovaries.

Estradiol (E2) is the dominant oestrogen in the body during a woman's childbearing years. During this time, there is a lot of Estradiol in your blood system. This hormone is produced mainly in your ovaries.

Estriol (E3) is the oestrogen of pregnancy as it is responsible for the growth of the placenta. Estriol promotes fertility, fetal growth and development, and it prepares your breasts for breastfeeding. When you are not pregnant, there is very little Estriol in your body – it is almost undetectable.

Oestrogen helps in the production of serotonin. If there is less oestrogen in your body, the amount of serotonin production also decreases. Consequently, this can affect your moods as the lack of serotonin puts you at risk of depression. A matter of concern during the menopause is that there is less oestrogen to promote healthy bone development. When oestrogen levels fall, bone loss begins to happen. Sometimes, this can lead to osteoporosis, a condition where bones become thin and fragile. Another concern is the health of the heart.

Oestrogen acts as a vital aid in keeping your blood vessels healthy. Without the protection that oestrogen helps to provide, there can be an increased level of inflammation in your blood vessels. There is also a decreased level of control over your cholesterol levels. Consequently, after you reach the menopause, you have an increased risk of developing heart disease.

When we are young girls, oestrogen is critical to start our periods. During our adult years, oestrogen aids us during pregnancy. When we are middle-aged, we can feel the benefits of having stronger bones and good heart health. As a woman goes into the menopause, the effects of a lack of oestrogen become more pronounced. The vagina, uterus, and breasts change, the vaginal walls become thinner, the lining of the uterus may increase, and you stop menstruating. When the menopause arrives, oestrogen production slows to a bare minimum. The sign that we used to look for, our period, is no longer there to help indicate the level of oestrogen in our body. Hence, we need to carefully observe our symptoms so that we decide whether to take supplements to replace the lack of oestrogen in our system.

Progesterone in Your Body

Progesterone is another critical hormone that gets the uterus ready for a fertilised egg and helps to maintain a successful and healthy pregnancy in the early stages. Reductions in progesterone also affect your menstrual periods. As your reproductive system stops the process of ovulation, your body stops producing progesterone. As a result, periods can become heavier and more extended during the perimenopause. Progesterone is closely tied with oestrogen because it helps with a woman's menstrual cycle. The part of your ovary that produces progesterone is called the corpus luteum. It develops from the follicle that is left behind when an egg leaves the ovary for fertilisation. The crucial role of progesterone is to prepare the lining of the uterus for the fertilised egg. If an egg is fertilised, you do not menstruate, but when there is no fertilisation, the corpus luteum dissolves, and your progesterone levels drop.

Progesterone is also produced in small amounts by the ovaries and adrenal glands. Progesterone is responsible for the growth of breast tissue, and it is also responsible for preparing your breasts for milk production and lactation.

Progesterone also plays a role in fertility, in particular, the development of a healthy thickening of your uterus lining. If there isn't enough progesterone in your body, the lining of the uterus will be thin, making it hard for a fertilised egg to attach itself. With the lack of progesterone during the menopause, your breasts may become sensitive, but it's mostly the lack of oestrogen that will make a difference during the menopause. There is some evidence that the lack of progesterone also plays a part in our moods. The signs of low progesterone are as follows:

- Irregular menstrual cycle.
- Mood changes (anxiety or depression)
- Headaches or migraines.
- Weight gain.
- Decreased sex drive.
- Mood swings (depression).
- PMS severity.

- Breast tenderness.
- Fibrocystic breasts.
- Fibroids.
- Gallbladder problems.
- Uterine bleeding.

Not all these symptoms will happen to you during the menopause. However, it is a good idea to be aware of them in case these symptoms start to affect your daily life, and it is necessary to see a doctor.

Testosterone in Your Body

Testosterone is a vital male sex hormone that is also produced by the ovaries in small amounts. It is a companion of oestrogen as it helps with the growth and repair of the female reproductive system, bone mass, and behaviour. Some symptoms of low testosterone include fatigue, increased weight gain, loss of bone and muscle loss, cognitive dysfunction, a reduction in libido and a lack of general energy. Although there is minimal testosterone production in a woman's body, adding testosterone can be a game-changer during the menopause. Treatments for regaining testosterone in the body have been around since 1936. Here are some benefits of testosterone treatments:

- Increased energy levels.
- A stronger feeling of well-being.
- Reduced breast sensitivity.
- Increased sexual desire.
- Better sexual sensitivity.
- Improved orgasms.

Testosterone is primarily understood as a vital hormone in the male body; however, testosterone is also an essential hormone for the female body. Testosterone helps the body to maintain a strong level of muscle and bone mass. Furthermore, testosterone also contributes to a woman's sex drive. Testosterone is at a peak level when a woman is in her twenties; however, after this peak of production, testosterone starts to drop, and it is at half the level when a woman begins the menopause. The good news is that testosterone production does not stop after the menopause; it is still produced in both the adrenal glands and the ovaries.

What Will Happen During the Medical Examination?

A woman needs to be seen regularly by either her GP or her gynaecologist. Sometimes women hesitate to see a gynaecologist because they are too busy, afraid, embarrassed or feel they have already seen them enough in the past (during pregnancies or for birth control needs). As the physical and psychological changes of the menopause occur, the symptoms may cause you enough concern to visit your doctor. Of course, the burning question will be when the last date of your period was. Moreover, there will be a medical exam undertaken to help your doctor assess the situation. As you have reached the menopause, there are concerns to be considered and addressed. Your doctor will be looking at the general health of your uterus, vagina, and cervix, evaluating how your bladder is working and examining the overall health of your fallopian tubes and ovaries. Overall, your pelvic exam is important because your doctor needs to rule out the risks of certain cancers because your risk increases as you age. Early detection is especially important and could save your life. Yes, you will still need pelvic exams. However, in the USA, after the age of sixty-five, if you've had three negative results in the past ten years, you can stop getting pelvic exams.

What to Ask your Doctor About the Menopause

Your doctor is a valuable resource when you are trying to understand the menopause. It's vital to feel confident when you go to see your doctor. Confidence allows you to ask questions that will help your doctor to treat many symptoms of the menopause, which are interrupting your daily routine. After your doctor has completed the examination, they may move on to a discussion about the best treatment plan for your circumstances. There are medications and therapy that may be prescribed to help alleviate the symptoms of the menopause. These include antidepressants, vaginal lubricants, Hormone Replacement Therapy (HRT) and Tibolone (like HRT). Hormone Replacement Therapy is a proven solution for relieving some of the most severe menopausal symptoms, but just how healthy is Hormone Replacement Therapy? I will discuss Hormone Replacement Therapy in more detail in chapter five. Hormone Replacement Therapy is usually prescribed in tablets, skin patches or gels.

Fourteen Vital Questions You Need to Discuss with Your Doctor

1. Are there medications that can ease some of my menopause symptoms?
2. Are there any lifestyle changes that I can make to relieve the symptoms of the menopause?
3. Could my symptoms be unrelated to the menopause?
4. What are the advantages and disadvantages of Hormone Replacement Therapy?
5. What are the side effects of Hormone Replacement Therapy?
6. Will you be prescribing any medications that are not Food and Drug Administration (FDA) approved for the menopause symptoms?
7. What herbal or food supplements would you suggest?

8. Are these supplements good for me? Will they harm me?

9. What are the over-the-counter medications that will relieve my menopause symptoms?

10. What is my baseline risk for breast, endometrial or ovarian cancer and other types of cancer?

11. If I am at risk for certain cancers, how much will Hormone Replacement Therapy raise my risk?

12. What is the risk of other severe conditions like heart disease, stroke, dangerous blood clots?

13. What other medicines can deliver the same or near results of Hormone Replacement Therapy?

14. Are the symptoms affecting your daily routine to a point where you can't do the things you need or love to do?

Reaching the Postmenopause

The postmenopause is the final stage where your ovaries stop releasing eggs and consequently, you stop having your periods. To be in the postmenopause, you need to have gone twelve consecutive months without a period. You will continue to have symptoms of the menopause for four to five years, but these symptoms start getting less intense over time. Your body will still be changing as you experience the loss of oestrogen and progesterone. You can no longer get pregnant naturally, but you can have hormone therapy and IVF to assist you if you still want to try and conceive a child. You will be postmenopausal for the rest of your life. Although you may have felt depressed or moody during the perimenopause, you will start to feel better and ready to go on this new journey in your life.

Screenings for Your Health

Now is not the time to give up on caring for your body. It is crucial to get regular breast and cervical health screenings to make sure that your body is in great shape. In the UK, women are actively encouraged to attend routine breast cancer screenings. According to the National Health Service (NHS) guidelines, all women between the ages of fifty to seventy-one are invited for free routine screenings, every three years. If you are under fifty years old and in a high-risk group, you may also be eligible for breast screening. In addition, the cervix is still susceptible to abnormalities even though you have entered the postmenopause. It is recommended by healthcare professionals, that women between twenty-five and forty-five-years old attend cervical screenings every three years. If you are between fifty and sixty-four years old, you ideally need to participate in a screening every five years.

Chapter Summary

The menopause is the time when your menstrual cycle stops, and you are no longer ovulating. The amount of the hormone oestrogen within your body begins to decrease. Oestrogen is responsible for many functions in your body. When oestrogen diminishes, this produces many often unnerving and uncomfortable symptoms like hot flushes, night sweats, and weight gain. Your heart health, bone health, and your moods will be affected by the absence of oestrogen. Oestrogen is not the only hormone that changes during the menopause. The amount of testosterone and progestogen in your body also begins to vary. The absence of progestogen is one of the key catalysts of the menopause. It is a vital hormone in relation to aiding both the menstrual cycle and fertility. Testosterone is crucial to ensure the growth and repair of your body. It is essential to visit your gynaecologist during and after the menopause. In the next chapter, you will discover more about the signs and symptoms of the menopause.

Chapter Three: Managing the Menopause

The Symptoms of the Menopause

Hot flushes	Night sweats	Insomnia
Palpitations	Headaches	Aching joints, muscles and tendons
Irritability and mood swings	Anxiety and panic attacks	Poor concentration
Poor memory	Loss of sex drive	Vaginal dryness (discomfort during sex)
Itchy skin	Lightheadedness	Dizziness

Tingling in arms and legs	Burning sensation in mouth	Tinnitus
Breast tenderness	Shrinking breast size	Fatigue
Indigestions, diarrhoea, wind and bloating	Increase in allergies	Change in body odour
Bleeding gums	Changes in fingernails	Feelings of fear and dread

It's easy from the table above to see that many symptoms can overlap with other conditions such as fatigue, aching joints, irritability, and mood swings. A thorough check-up can rule out other conditions besides menopause.

In the modern world, health professionals take the place of family and guide women through the "change". In today's digital world, there is almost too much information. In the few minutes that you have for yourself, you try to get through all the information, but you are tired, and the words don't make much sense to you. It's good to be able to access case studies and medical reports, but who is there to interpret them for you?

This chapter will explore the physiological signs and symptoms of the menopause. You will not experience all the symptoms and signs of the menopause. Some women have a few, and some women barely have one. You may even have experienced a symptom and not realised it was connected to the menopause. So, don't panic! I will explain each symptom so that you have a clear understanding of it. This chapter will not outline specific drug treatments. It is always advised to consult your doctor for any medical treatments. They will be able to give you the most accurate advice and support based on your medical history and current circumstances.

The Symptoms of the Menopause – in More Detail

Hot flushes — Feel like you have a fever? Are you the

only one in the room that is on fire? The chances are that you are experiencing hot flushes. The heat from hot flushes takes over your body from head to toe. You tend to feel flushed, especially a redness on your face. Fifty per cent of women will experience hot flushes. Some women only experience them in certain situations, and others have them all the time. Hot flushes start during the perimenopause and go on through the menopause. Hot flushes are not a 24/7 type of symptom. Sometimes they only happen at night.

***Triggers*:** stress, caffeine, alcohol, spicy foods, tight clothing, heat, and cigarette smoke.

***Solutions*:** Hormone Replacement Therapy or natural alternatives.

***Night Sweats*—** It's night-time, and you have been sleeping for a few hours. You wake up to use the bathroom, feeling very uncomfortable and drenched in sweat. Even your pillow and sheets are wet. You've just experienced night sweats.

Solution: a chilled pillow filled with water, slow abdominal breathing exercises, exercise, walking, swimming, bicycling, dancing.

Fatigue — If you aren't sleeping because you have been having hot flushes and night sweats, it would be understandable that you are tired during the day. However, you can get a good night's rest and still feel this chronic tiredness. Your productivity goes down, and you have difficulty even doing the most straightforward task. This kind of fatigue starts to affect your relationships and your moods. Your stress is increased because you are so tired that you start falling behind in every aspect of your life.

Solution: moderate to high-intensity exercises (like yoga), a good sleep routine, a meditation break, a low thermostat setting at night, light dinners, drinking more water, limiting alcohol and caffeine, and following a healthy diet.

Memory lapses and foggy thinking — The good news about this symptom is that after the menopause, the fog will gently lift, and your memory will improve. However, during the menopause, you will have difficulty remembering things. You won't become an amnesiac; you'll "flush" forget information like your phone number or how many eggs you just cracked into the frying pan. Oestrogen and progesterone are thought to affect a woman's memory. So, the lack of these two hormones can impact how the brain works. Brain fog or memory lapses will go away in time.

Solutions: Taking a low dose of oestrogen or a combination of progestin can help. Hormone Replacement Therapy, a balanced diet, rest, exercise, and meditation may help.

Loss of libido (decreased level of sex drive) — At first, it was just because you were tired, but it's been a month, and you don't even miss sex. What is going on? Due to the menopause, you are fatigued and irritable. You have trouble just being kind to your partner during dinner, much less, during sex. It isn't just all in your head. Sex has become painful thanks to vaginal dryness. Even if you felt like having sex, it is just too painful to endure.

The decline of oestrogen in your body will have an impact on your vagina. During the menopause, the natural moisture of the vagina vanishes. Even the natural lubrication that you are used to will disappear. The dryness becomes a significant issue for having sex.

Solutions: Hormone Replacement Therapy, Vaginal oestrogen, Vaginal moisturisers, water-based lubricant before sex, avoiding douches, bubble baths, scented soaps, and lotions around sensitive areas. Your doctor will recommend over-the-counter medications to help you deal with vaginal dryness.

Urinary tract infections — You've rarely had urinary infections, but now they seem to be happening with some frequency. During the menopause, having a lower amount of oestrogen causes a change in vaginal bacteria.

Solutions: Hormone Replacement Therapy, Vaginal Oestrogen, antibiotics and natural remedies.

Bloating — This time it's the high levels of oestrogen that cause the trouble. You begin to feel like you are too full, and your belly is going to burst. Your stomach is swollen and tight and feels like a football. Just be patient, what goes up must come down. Your oestrogen levels will fall, and then you will have some relief from bloating.

Solutions: Stay hydrated by drinking plenty of fresh water, exercise regularly, avoid trigger foods, avoid carbonated drinks, don't chew gum, quit smoking, reduce salt intake, eat probiotics and eat smaller meals.

Mood swings — In chapter four, we will discuss what happens to your brain during the menopause. The neurotransmitters in your brain are affected by the ups and downs of your hormonal levels. Gamma-aminobutyric acid (GABA) and serotonin are two neurotransmitters that are known to have an impact on our moods. Too little serotonin and you are susceptible to depression. Further, the neurotransmitter that is not working well can cause mood swings and irritability.

Solutions: If you feel that mood swings are affecting your ability to function in everyday life, please consult your doctor for a referral to specialised health professionals.

Anxiety — You may have an increase in anxiety for the same reasons that you have a mood swing, i.e. lack of neurotransmitters in the brain. Also, you might be disturbed due to the mood swings and are not able to feel relaxed and calm.

Solutions: See your doctor for a referral to a mental health professional, as they may prescribe antidepressants.

Depression — Again, the lack of neurotransmitters due to fluctuating oestrogen can cause clinical depression. Trying to adjust to other symptoms of the menopause like mood swings and other symptoms can also lead a person to experience feelings of distress.

Solutions: See your doctor. They can evaluate your depression and refer you to a therapist, psychiatrist or counsellor. Depression and lack of serotonin in your brain— your doctor will recommend clonidine (a high blood pressure medicine) or antidepressants. The reason for antidepressants is to replace some of the serotonin that might be diminishing in your brain.

Hair Loss and Thinning — Low levels of oestrogen impair the growth of hair and hair follicles, so your hair gets dry and brittle. You might find a lot of hair falling out onto your brush or when you shampoo your hair. Forty per cent of women experience hair loss during the menopause.

Solutions: Reduce stress, exercise, eat well, hydrate, nourish follicles by using a special shampoo, and talk to your doctor.

Brittle Nails — Lack of oestrogen makes nails brittle, dry, and easy to break.

Solution: Pamper your nails, quit smoking, enhance your diet, protect your hands, and moisturise.

Itchy Skin — Decreasing levels of oestrogen at the beginning of the perimenopause and the menopause affect collagen production. Low levels of collagen cause thin, dry, itchy skin and the loss of collagen makes your skin appear older.

Solutions: Avoid hot baths or showers, dry your skin gently after bathing, avoid scratching, use scent-free skin care, reduce alcohol and nicotine intake, wear soft and loose fabrics, avoid strong sunlight and stay well hydrated. Reduce stress, apply a cold and wet cloth or ice pack to the skin, oatmeal baths, moisturise and use cooling agents like menthol or calamine lotion. Please see a dermatologist if you feel your symptoms are getting out of control.

Sleep Disorders including Insomnia — It's a toss-up as to whether you can't sleep because of the issues that happen in midlife or if the hormonal fluctuations are causing you to lose sleep. Insomnia, sleep disorders, breathing, night sweats, and anxiety are thought to occur during the menopause. Insomnia may be a reaction to night sweats, hot flushes, anxiety, and panic disorders. Low levels of oestrogen caused by the onset of the menopause may also be linked to the inability to sleep properly.

Solutions: Try to maintain good sleep hygiene, exercise regularly (but not just before going to sleep), avoid excessive caffeine and alcohol, maintain a healthy diet, get some sunshine (melatonin), try cognitive-behavioural therapy to help with troublesome thoughts, and avoid taking naps during the day. Please consult your doctor if you experience sleep apnoea.

Dizziness — Do you feel dizzy for an extended period? Does dizziness impair your daily routine? This might be happening due to the menopause. The frequency and length of the dizzy spells may lead to falling or not being able to walk on your own.

Solutions: Lying down and closing your eyes until you feel better, acupuncture, staying hydrated, reduce stress, limiting alcohol and caffeine, getting restful sleep.

Weight Gain — As if you didn't have enough trouble staying trim before, the menopause will cause you to gain extra weight and make it harder to lose it again. Muscle and lean body mass diminish, and fat redistributes itself and gathers in the abdomen.

***Solutions*:** Exercise regularly through the menopause to build your muscles back up and jump-start your metabolic rate.

Digestive Problems — Routine abdominal pain and discomfort happen when digestion slows. When oestrogen is absent, there is no aid to help the body keep cortisol levels at a minimum. If your levels of cortisol get too high, digestion is slowed, leaving you to feel bloated or constipated.

***Solutions*:** (See bloating), also consider dietary changes such as eating more whole grains, bran, raspberries, pears, apples, peas, broccoli, legumes, nuts, and seeds. Try pelvic floor exercises. Please consult your doctor if you experience pain, nausea, vomiting, the inability to pass gas, or extreme bloating.

Muscle Tension — Do you feel your muscles tighten in your neck, back, and shoulders? The menopause can bring about soreness, aches and stiffness.

Solution: Gentle massage, simple stretching exercises, good posture, reduce stress.

Headaches — The decrease in the production of oestrogen may cause women to have more frequent and intense headaches. Good news, the headaches go away or become less frequent after the perimenopause.

Solution: Keep a diary of things such as foods that trigger a migraine, eat meals at regular times, go to sleep and wake up at the same time each day, relax to avoid stress, try meditation, deep breathing and massages.

Incontinence — The reduction of oestrogen causes three types of incontinence:

1. **Urinary incontinence:** the internal muscles of the pelvic floor fail.

2. **Overflow incontinence:** the lack of any sensation that your bladder is full.

3. **Accidental urination:** the brain fails to recognise

that your bladder is full.

***Solutions*:** See your doctor for tests to rule out more serious issues, keep a bladder diary of the details of your incontinence (what you drink, when do you have the urge to urinate, the level of urine you produce, and the number of times you were incontinent). Try pelvic floor exercises, incontinence pads, keep a self-care pack including a spare pair of underwear, wipes, pads, and deodorant in your bag.

Burning Tongue — The variations in your oestrogen levels can cause a metallic taste in your mouth. A burning sensation can happen on your tongue, lips, gums and other spots in your mouth. The causes are still unknown.

***Solution*s:** See your doctor who will investigate the issue further. They may suggest cognitive behaviour therapy.

Allergies — Your body's immune system becomes compromised by hormonal fluctuations that occur during the menopause. When this happens, you can become more sensitive to allergens. You can experience mild to severe reactions. Think rashes, itchy eyes, sneezing, dizziness, cramping, and swelling.

***Solutions*:** Over-the-counter-medications for specific allergies. See your doctor if you are having respiratory issues such as asthma.

Body Odour Change — Low levels of oestrogen cause false messages to be sent to the hypothalamus. When this happens, the hypothalamus tells the body it is hot, and there is an increase in perspiration. This hyper perspiration changes the natural scent of a woman. Increased body odour and sweating generally subside over time.

***Solutions*:** lifestyle changes, rethinking your diet, reducing stress, being prepared, keeping deodorant in your purse.

Osteoporosis — Oestrogen prevents your bones from undertaking the process of bone resorption. During the menopause, your oestrogen levels drop, and you may undergo loss of bone mass density. As a result, your bones are in peril of becoming brittle and weak. Osteoporosis is a degenerative bone disorder that menopausal women are at risk of developing because of a lack of oestrogen.

Solution: Weight-bearing exercises, eating a balanced diet rich in vitamins and minerals from plant sources. Please see your doctor for further advice and support, if you think you may have Osteoporosis. Your health care professional will be able to offer advice regarding a lifestyle change to help you deal with the condition (exercise regularly, eat a healthy diet, get sunlight, and stop smoking and drinking alcohol). Further, they may prescribe some calcium or vitamin D supplements.

Tingling Extremities — Your extremities may feel like they are burning, or like an insect is biting you. It feels like your arms, hands, legs and feet are tingling non-stop.

Solutions: A balanced diet, hydration, exercise, a good night's sleep, Hormone Replacement Therapy, Omega-3 fatty acids, Vitamin B, Vitamin C Vitamin E, phytoestrogens, magnesium, potassium, exercise, fighting fatigue, good posture, massages; avoid saturated fats, cigarettes, caffeine and alcohol.

Electric Shock Sensation — Brief feelings of electric shock due to low oestrogen levels can occur throughout the body. It usually comes before a hot flush. These sensations can be hard to experience. Electric sensations may pass suddenly through areas of the head, like feeling a zap or surge moving just under the skin.

Solutions: Lifestyle changes, alternative medicine, and medications.

Difficulty Concentrating — The inability to focus or to concentrate can be a sign of the perimenopause or the menopause. Decreasing levels of progesterone also affect memory and focus. Lack of sleep and mood swings can also add to the feeling of confusion.

Solutions: A well-balanced diet, restful sleep, exercise, both physical and mental (puzzles, crosswords, socialising). See a doctor if memory issues are so severe that it results in neglecting personal hygiene, being unable to name familiar objects, or having difficulty following directions. You doctor may also recommend Menopausal Hormone Therapy (MHT), low dose oestrogen or a combo of oestrogen and progestin.

Irregular Heartbeat — The decrease of oestrogen in your body may cause overstimulation of the nervous and circulatory systems. This resulting overstimulation can trigger an irregular heartbeat, palpitations, and arrhythmias.

Solution: If you have these symptoms, consult your doctor at once.

Breast Pain — Before the menopause, oestrogen and progesterone are produced in the correct amounts. This allows the breasts to keep their form and shape. However, during the menopause, these hormones are absent. The breasts are no longer able to keep their shape and begin to fall. Hormonal fluctuations cause sharp pains and tenderness in your breasts. One or both breasts can be affected. There can also be tenderness in each breast. The good news is that once you've gone through the menopause, the pain usually goes away.

Solution: See your doctor who may recommend oral contraceptives and cut back on caffeine.

Joint Pain — Joint pain may happen due to declining oestrogen levels. Specifically, inflammation may occur that causes this pain. Women will feel the following symptoms:

- Aching or tingling in fingers.
- Tightness in the hips.
- Soreness in the knees.
- Swelling of various joints.

This inflammation can lead to arthritis. Declining bone density can also cause joint pain or soreness.

Solution: Eat anti-inflammatory rich foods, exercise regularly, manage your weight, hydrate with plenty of water, use ice packs to reduce swelling and reduce your stress levels. See a doctor to rule out other causes of inflammation and for advice regarding the use of taking magnesium glycinate, glucosamine, and chondroitin supplements.

Chapter Summary

There are about thirty-five different symptoms associated with the menopause. Most of the symptoms have solutions that can be applied to provide much needed relief. It is a rare thing for a woman to have all thirty-five symptoms. Most women will only experience a few of the symptoms. The symptoms of menopause can range from minimal to excessive. In the next chapter, you will discover more about optimal brain health during the menopause.

Chapter Four: What Happens to My Brain During the Menopause?

In the course of this chapter, we will look behind the scenes of some key menopausal symptoms. We will delve deeper into the mental and emotional symptoms you may face during the menopause. These include crying, confusion, mental fog, forgetfulness and irritation. During mid-life, you might feel that everything you know and are used too is changing in your life. Instead of your parents taking care of you; you are taking care of them. The kids are grown up; you start worrying about how they will survive on their own. Your job changes and your new bosses all seem to have just graduated from nursery school. Your mind is always in a whirlwind. You are supposed to be thinking about work, you're thinking about your family, and when you are with your family, you are thinking about your job.

On top of that, your brain feels like it is in a fog.

You start to forget so many things that now you can't make it without an assistant's help: real or artificial help like Syrie (Apple's AI), Alexia (Amazon's AI) or Cortana (Windows AI). Finally, the date you most want to forget: your birthday comes around more quickly than ever, you feel you might as well say you are a hundred and work from there. It has been weeks, months, or even years since you felt one hundred per cent mentally or physically. So precisely what is wrong?

Society, in general, sends the message that without oestrogen, you will grow old, wither, and die because your body doesn't have the hormones that it needs to function. How many dynamic women do you know who are in their mid-life and are happy and flourishing? Before you run to your gynaecologist for hormone replacement, let's look at what exactly is happening to your body and mind and what you can do about it. Like women before you, it's possible to conquer the emotional and mental effects of the menopause.

It is often thought that a cognitive change during the menopause is imagined; however, a study cited in Prevention magazine illustrates the fact that menopausal women are not imagining the mental changes they are going through. In this study, two thousand three hundred women were observed over four years, and the researchers found that the fluctuating levels of oestrogen caused a drop in a person's cognitive abilities. This fluctuation also affected the participant's moods and emotions. When it came to measuring a woman's processing speed, verbal and working memory, there were declines in the menopausal study group. When these women were given the oestrogen hormone to supplement what their bodies weren't producing, their cognitive skills increased.

A Storm in a Teacup

It starts with the perimenopause; the mood swings, depression, and even tantrums. Maybe you feel as if you are slowly going crazy and that crying, yelling, and anxiety is your new normal. It is normal to feel weepy during the menopause and studies have found that women who have had severe premenstrual syndrome are more likely to have emotional issues due to the menopause. Many women endure episodes of anxiety, panic attacks and nervousness. According to the North American Menopause Society (NAMS), twenty-three per cent of women experience mood swings before, during and after menopause. Besides, up to seventy per cent of women reported they had to deal with irritability during the menopausal. The NAMS caution that woman with a history of depression or other mental issues are at a higher risk of developing emotional episodes during the menopause. These symptoms occur where there is a fluctuation in your hormone levels. There is evidence to suggest that low oestrogen levels interfere with the production of serotonin, insulin metabolism, and cholesterol. Menopausal women tend to be in a phase of their life where lots of significant changes coincide. A drop-in oestrogen levels seems to magnify what is going on. It's not so much that you are overreacting or being picky; your brain is just experiencing new changes due to the menopause.

So just what is happening within your body to cause such a high level of mental and emotional upheaval? First, there are receptors for oestrogen and progesterone in the ovaries and other organs. Since your oestrogen level is diminishing, your whole body takes notice, especially your brain. So, mood-regulating chemicals like serotonin and endorphins are affected. Specifically, the lack of oestrogen affects the production of these essential brain chemicals. Consequently, the delicate biochemistry of the brain is disrupted. Now, your ovaries, if you still have them, are trying hard to produce oestrogen but they are out of balance. Some days they produce too much oestrogen, and other days they produce very little. It is a wonder that a woman doesn't lose her mind entirely.

Oestrogen hinders the body's ability to deal with serotonin and norepinephrine. A lack of these vital hormones in the body could also be linked to an increased risk of depression. Risk factors for an emotional issue during the menopause include complicated relationships with loved ones, an excessive amount of daily stress and an unsatisfactory living situation. In addition, during the menopause, the brain has been found by researchers to have high levels of monoamine oxidase A (MAO-A). This brain protein is linked to depression in women entering menopause. Critical signs of depression include extreme sadness, loss of interest in activities, no motivation to do the things you used to love, difficulty sleeping, and the inability to concentrate. It may be tempting for some to self-medicate with alcohol and drugs (this is never a wise option to consider under any circumstances). If you feel any of these signs apply to you, please don't be afraid of seeking professional help and guidance.

It's vital to remember that you are not the first woman to go through this. Everybody is different, and it's normal that you will experience 'the change' in your unique way. If you haven't lost your mind due to the menopause, you are just fine. It doesn't mean that any minute you are going to go nuts. It just means that your body is behaving in a way that isn't outlandish. Who knows, maybe your ovaries are hardworking and prone to perfectionism and produce the right amount of oestrogen. There are simple strategies you can utilise to boost and improve both your moods and your memory. We will discuss these strategies later in the chapter.

It's difficult to imagine the emotional surges and the forgetfulness that occurs during the menopause. These symptoms are genuine. However, you can play an active role in compensating for these high emotions caused by the irregular distribution of hormones within your body. There is currently a great deal of research being undertaken to understand how positive thoughts affect our brain. When you are in emotional distress, analyse your life for a moment and think about your level of stress. Remember, this is a no judgement. If the menopause has driven you to the edge, that is okay. Understandably, you are under a lot of stress because of this.

Stress is not something that you hold onto but instead something that you work to release. Some people think that you can stand in the middle of your kitchen and say, *"I'm done with my stress"*, and it all goes away. However, it's not as simple as just wishing your stress away. You are going to have to take some active measures to get rid of this stress. Many women who are regular smokers use cigarettes as a way of trying to combat stress. The nicotine in cigarettes is a sedative, but it is also a stimulant. If you are already experiencing irritability, depression and mood swings, smoking will augment these feelings and even make you feel worse than before. If you are currently smoking and want to quit see your general practitioner for help.

There are many positive steps you can take to manage stress. Your smartphone is a perfect time manager. Not into the digital world? A pen and paper to-do-list can also do the trick. Post-it notes can be bought anywhere and are a great way to remind yourself to do things. Choose a bright colour you love and put notes everywhere you need to remember something. It doesn't have to be dramatic, keeping a notebook on your desk or in your purse can do the trick. Putting lists on your phone or a memo pad is a system that has been proven to be successful. It's not just about listing things to scratch off as done. It's also about organising the project or problem that you must solve. Often, when you must write a list, you are forced to look at the situation. The process leads to improved lateral thinking and problem-solving abilities.

Your Support Network

Even if you are the only adult in your home, it is good to give your children things to do. It helps them feel better about themselves. Along with delegating, try and make a promise to be kind to yourself. Since your hormones are fluctuating, there are going to be days that you feel good and days where you feel awful. Use the positive days to give your daily tasks two hundred per cent. If you are the sort of person that is confident talking about your feelings, a support group is a great way to cut down on stress. Check if any formal group meets at your local community centre. Alternatively, your support group may be a group phone call with other women going through similar experiences.

Friends who will listen when you need to talk about your menopause journey are so valuable. Cultivate friendships that are supportive and positive. If you have very little time in your day, there are support groups online or forums for discussions about the menopause. If you are a night owl, you might find some support groups in a country that is in a time zone that compliments your schedule. The internet knows no geographical boundaries and women go through the menopause no matter their nationality or location.

Make Time for Exercise and Sleep Well

In a world where you feel that is everything is topsy turvy, it's good to know that doing something physical can make the world stop spinning. You can join an exercise group or exercise in the privacy of your own home. Moreover, there are even chair exercises that you can do at work. Whatever your style, moving your body helps to produce mood-enhancing endorphins. Have some fun trying out different types of physical exercises. It's always easier to stick to an exercise routine if you enjoy what you are doing. Many women find the practice of yoga or tai chi to be a beneficial addition to their exercise routine. Daily meditation has also proven to be helpful. When you have a grounded "centre" and become mindful, you are less overwhelmed and find it easier to deal with your emotional issues.

Although insomnia is known to happen during the menopause, you can try to practice good bedtime habits. There is some evidence to suggest that the use of electrical devices and prolonged exposure to blue light can disrupt your sleep cycle. There are steps you can take to reduce this unwanted disruption to your vital need for sleep. It is wise to turn off and remove addictive devices such as laptops and mobiles from your sleep space. Try to set a firm rule not to use electric devices for at least an hour before going to bed. If you are at all concerned about the possible effects of blue light, there are extensions you can add to your phone and laptop to reduce blue light and special blue light blocking glasses you can wear at home. However, it's crucial that you find a solution that soothes you and that you enjoy building into your nightly routine. For example, you could watch black and white movies and take bubble baths before you go to sleep. Try to think outside the box, and you will find a bedtime routine that works for you. The critical thing is to make the time for the routine. Don't skip the routine and expect to sleep the minute you jump into bed if you have insomnia.

Eating and Drinking for Peace of Mind

The jury isn't out yet on the connection between food and serotonin. Tryptophan, an amino acid, can help your body to create serotonin. Serotonin stimulates your mood, and there is a link between the lack of serotonin in the body and a decreased level of mood. Consequently, adding serotonin-supporting foods to your diet is an excellent way to help you achieve a healthy level of serotonin. Examples of foods with high levels of tryptophan include dairy, nuts, poultry, spinach and salmon. Tryptophan rich foods usually need to partner up with some carbohydrates to be effective. The body then breaks carbohydrates down into sugars that past into the bloodstream and cause a spike in your blood sugar levels. As a result, the pancreas produces insulin, and this makes it easier for amino acids like tryptophan to be absorbed. Mixing foods that are high in tryptophan with carbohydrates might put more serotonin in your bloodstream, creating an increase in serotonin. The downside is that amino acids compete with each other to be utilised by the brain, so there is a chance that you won't get that boost. However, you can have a better chance if you eat a healthy serving of tryptophan-rich foods with carbohydrates. Examples of healthy carbohydrates to add to your diet include vegetables, pulses, whole grains, nuts and seeds.

Eating isn't the only way to increase serotonin. Sunshine, positivity, and exercise can help improve your serotonin levels. Plus, exercising can help to chase away those blues. If you find yourself depressed or in a bad mood all the time, ask your doctor if you need a serotonin supplement. During the menopause, your body becomes depleted of certain chemicals and causes changes in the brain. If you find that you are a regular at your local coffee house or your favourite drinks are caffeinated soda or tea, be aware that caffeine is a stimulant. Caffeine is known to play havoc with your mood swings. Also, caffeine can disturb your sleep cycle. Consider buying decaffeinated tea from your local supermarket. If caffeine is a hard habit to break, consider only drinking caffeinated beverages in the morning and having no further caffeinated drinks after lunch.

There is a way to fight back and decrease the

effects of the menopause. It's so important to exercise and add more healthy foods to your diet. These simple steps help to increase the levels of vital chemicals. The menopause can be looked at as an alert to take better care of yourself and become proactive in maintaining your health.

Seek Professional Help

Even though there has not been an official link or discovery, there is still evidence that the menopause may cause insomnia and mood swings. If the mood swings of the menopause have overwhelmed you, please seek professional help for further support and guidance. There may be questions over concerns that the menopause could impact the effects of mental illnesses. If you have bipolar disorder or other serious mental health issues such as schizophrenia, you may want to consult your mental health professional. Ask your doctor about your current medication plan. They will advise whether any change in your medication is needed, as there may be extra stress on your system during the menopause.

At the same time, as you reach the menopause, you may also be going through some very tough life changes. Often in midlife, we lose our parents or other special people who are very close to us. A major traumatic event such as the loss of family members or close friends can trigger a depressive episode, and it can decrease oestrogen in your body. This decrease may be enough to trigger depression or make it more intense. Health care professionals will understand the emotional upheavals you have experienced. The health care professionals will be able to address your psychological condition. They will work together with you to create the best treatment plan for your circumstances. So, don't feel like you are going crazy; remember that your body is changing, and this will affect your mental health. Some alternatives to consider with your health care professional are:

- Hormone therapy.
- Selective serotonin reuptake inhibitors (SSRIs).
- Complementary alternative medicines (CAM).
- Low dose birth control pills.

- Black Cohosh.
- Deep breathing.
- Soy.
- Acupuncture.
- Mind-body therapies (yoga, tai chi, and meditation).

Many women turn to herbal remedies such as St. John's Wort for help with various emotional issues. It is always wise to consult your doctor before trying new herbal remedies. Certain supplements and treatments may interfere with your current prescription medications.

Sexual Health

There are specific symptoms of the menopause that make it difficult to have sex. Also, there are certain negative mood states, like depression or irritability, that predispose a woman not to want to have sex with her partner. Low Libido, known as hypoactive sexual desire disorder (HSDD), happens to some women during the menopause. The symptoms of hypoactive sexual desire disorder include a dry vagina, loss of vaginal secretions, pelvic pain and discomfort during sex, an inability to reach orgasm, and a loss of desire. Hypoactive sexual desire disorder is the most common sexual problem found in women going through the menopause. Hypoactive sexual desire disorder is directly related to both the perimenopause and menopause. Hypoactive sexual desire disorder can occur no matter the partner, situation, or sexual activity. The combination of physical pain and emotional difficulties can be addressed with hormones, medications and counselling. Oestrogen therapy can help improve and support the walls of the vagina and vaginal dryness. Oestrogen can be applied using a cream to relieve discomfort and weakness in the vaginal walls. Testosterone can improve hypoactive sexual desire disorder by helping the brain cells in the limbic system that influence emotion. Testosterone can also improve the condition of the genital tissue of the labia, clitoris and the "G" spot.

Although there are many causes of sexual dysfunction during or after the menopause, there are many solutions. They range from medical or psychological therapies to self-help activities that you can try on your own. Support and excellent communication with your partner are an excellent start to improving your sex life. Interventions like sex therapy or couples counselling can also help you overcome your sexual concerns. It is not uncommon to encounter multiple physical and emotional issues concerning your sex life. Sometimes, vaginal dryness and fragile vaginal tissue is the reason a woman does not feel like engaging in sexual activity. When this is the case, vaginal oestrogen may be prescribed by your doctor. This type of oestrogen comes in the form of a cream, tablet or ring. Some women, when the menopause occurs, find themselves divorced, widowed, or single. It is necessary to remember to still use caution when having intercourse and protect against STDs. Moreover, the fragile vaginal tissue in untreated menopausal women is more susceptible to infection.

The Brain During the Menopause

Although there are more than thirty-five physical symptoms connected to the menopause, mental symptoms are just as important to consider. When experiencing these emotional symptoms, women may be told that it is only a figment of their imagination. They might be diagnosed with a mood disorder and given medication that is not appropriate for their symptoms. It's vital to understand the emotional toll of the menopause. It allows individuals to become active and knowledgeable participants in their mental health treatment. Before we knew about serotonin and its role in depression, the sometimes-debilitating emotional symptoms of the menopause were thought to be a dramatic exaggeration on the part of a woman. Today we know differently, and you have many resources at your fingertips. Be mindful of mood swings and seek appropriate care whether it be with a psychiatrist, therapist, psychiatric nurse practitioner, or counsellor. Here are four simple tips you can use to help you from becoming overwhelmed by the menopause:

1. Postpone making tough decisions until your emotions have stabilised. Try speaking to a friend or family member to help you get some perspective on your current situation.

2. Incorporate enjoyable social events into your weekly routine (exercising, attending a sporting event, going to the cinema).

3. Large tasks can be broken down into smaller tasks and prioritised so that you can handle things better.

4. Make a promise to be kind to yourself and keep in mind that your emotional and physical symptoms will get better with time.

Chapter Summary

The menopause does not just affect us physically. Mental and emotional changes are also taking place during the menopause. Specifically, a lack of oestrogen leads to a disruption in the level of serotonin within the brain. This disruption is responsible for mood swings and depression. Some women are affected so severely by these mood swings; it affects their daily routines. During the menopause, a woman's sexuality might also be affected. The change in sexual desire can be treated with new medication or therapies. If the menopause affects you emotionally and sexually in a significant way, it is appropriate for you to seek medical attention to correct this situation.

Chapter Five: What are the Pros and Cons of HRT?

Many women look for relief from the symptoms of the menopause, especially when the symptoms have become so severe, they interrupt daily activities. Gynaecological endocrinology is the study of hormones produced by the ovaries, or those hormones that influence the function of the ovaries. Hormones are steroid and protein messengers that are in our blood and pass between cells. Various glands secrete hormones within the body and brain. Hormones are released in the thymus, pancreas, and ovaries. They are also released in the hypothalamus and the pituitary gland in the brain. These hormones are responsible for keeping our cells functioning properly. The most common glands in a woman that secrete hormones and give directions to the cells are the ovaries. There are three essential hormones produced by the ovaries; Progesterone, Testosterone and Oestrogen.

As previously stated, oestrogen is the name of a group of hormones: Estradiol, Estrone and Estriol. When there are no longer any eggs in the ovary, oestrogen (produced by the ovary) levels fall substantially. The cells that depend on oestrogen no longer function normally. When the ovary no longer secretes oestrogen, there are physical changes and symptoms which put a woman in distress. When this happens, hormone replacement therapy can be administered to restore cell function and help cure the symptoms that have occurred.

What is HRT (Hormone Replacement Therapy)?

Due to the advancement of endocrinology during the twentieth century, women found relief for their symptoms through hormone replacement therapy. In the early part of the twentieth century, oestrogen and progesterone were singled out to be the most important hormones to replace in a woman's body. Many synthetic forms for these hormones have since been manufactured. There are several types of hormone therapies. These therapies include oestrogen (Estradiol, Estrone and Estriol) only therapies, oestrogen combined with Progestogen (Progestin US), or Progestogen-only treatments.

The therapy works by replacing vital hormones that are missing inside a woman's body. When you replace a hormone, there is a "messenger" in the body that will enable the cells to carry out their function or "work". When the body has the correct level of various hormones, it keeps the body stable and in balance. In the 1960s, the oral contraceptive was introduced, also known as the birth control pill, and doctors realised that they could also prescribe the pill to help women with their menopause symptoms. In the last fifty years, oral hormone replacement therapy has become user-friendly and easy to prescribe and take.

Any woman experiencing extreme symptoms of the perimenopause or menopause can receive hormone replacement therapy. Some conditions may prevent you from being a candidate for HRT. If you have had a stroke or heart disease, a history of blood clots, endometrial, breast or ovarian cancer, dementia, gallbladder disease, vision loss due to a blood clot in your eye, liver problems, or high blood pressure, your doctor may caution you from having HRT.

Things to Discuss with your Doctor

The chances are that you will have some symptoms of the menopause. If those symptoms are extreme, you will be looking for relief. HRT could be the relief that you need, but what about the risks? HRT has been linked to cancer, but overall the increased risk is small. It is essential to discuss with your doctor the severity of your symptoms. Together you and your doctor can assess the risks and benefits of each treatment. They can also create the most effective treatment plan for you. You and your doctor can decide precisely the hormone that can help to decrease or cure the extreme menopause symptoms that you are experiencing.

HRT Regimens

To decide whether to have hormone replacement treatments, you must consider the different regimens of HRT.

There are three main types of HRT regimens, such as:

- Oestrogen and/or Progesterone.
- Progestin/Progestogen.
- Specific Oestrogen Receptor Modulators (SERM's).

To decide whether to have hormone replacement treatments, you must consider the different regimens of HRT. You must consider whether the hormones are natural or synthetic. Also, you need to know whether therapy will be prescribed in low or high doses and how it will be administered. Specifically, will it be administered orally, transdermally (above the skin), subdermally (implant under the skin), or transbuccally (absorbed by the cheek or mouth)? Another thing to take into consideration is if there will be other hormones administered such as Progestogen, Testosterone, or Dehydroepiandrosterone sulfate (DHEAS) that will be added to the oestrogen.

The goal of HRT is to give the patient the hormones that they are missing. HRT regimens help to manage the symptoms of the menopause. Specifically, a patient is being treated for a symptom that has become so extreme they are having trouble functioning. Consequently, they will be given a hormone that will relieve this symptom. HRT can be designed to be specific for the woman who is taking it. For example, patient may be suffering for hot flushes, night sweats, and insomnia. Since the symptoms of the menopause are unique to each woman, it makes sense to design therapy around the needs of each woman. Your regimen will be adjusted to your needs. The way you receive HRT is varied and flexible. There will be a choice between a bioidentical or synthetic hormone, and you will have the option of how you take this hormone. For example, the following considerations are taken when prescribing a therapy:

- **Oestrogen** is given to protect the bones and the brain. HRT has also been found to decrease the risk of heart attacks, hypertension and dementia in the post-menopausal years. It also helps to control and diminish mood swings and depression during the perimenopause. Oestrogen is known to influence heart health and maintaining optimal levels of serotonin in the brain. It also helps maintain the moisture and elasticity of the vagina (potential better sexual enjoyment). Post-menopausal women have symptoms of the skin losing its suppleness and firmness due to the loss of Estradiol (oestrogen), but the introduction of HRT causes the skin to improve. The skin cells of the vagina and clitoris are helped to become supple and firm once again.

- **Progestogen** is given to protect the uterus, in particular, the endometrial lining. Breakthrough bleeding can occur when the lining of the uterus becomes very thick. Consequently, it outgrows its blood supply and the cells on the surface of the lining die. This exposes fragile blood vessels. The resulting breakdown leads to heavy bleeding. HRT can help by adding progesterone to oppose the oestrogen that is being added to your body.

- **Testosterone** is used to improve and enhance the sex organs, the brain and the libido, along with muscle tone.

- **SERMs** reduce the risk of osteoporotic fractures caused by the weakening of bones. SERM's have also been known to decrease the risk of breast cancer.

Some Popular Forms of HRT

Oral therapy is the most popular form of HRT. However, there is a problem with the rapid breakdown of progesterone and oestrogen by enzymes in the gut and liver. This doesn't leave the correct level of both hormones to be released successfully into the bloodstream. Consequently, transdermal therapy has been created to solve this problem. A small patch is applied to your arm or anywhere else on the body, and it continually releases the hormone for up to a week. Estradiol, one of the hormones grouped under the term oestrogen, has an oral bioidentical. Although a new way to receive this hormone, it has been linked to problems in the liver. Estradiol is broken done too quickly in the gut and liver, which does not let enough Estradiol get into the bloodstream. Also, there is a surge in liver production of clotting factors and a rise in levels of sex hormone-binding globulin.

Systemic hormone therapy allows a hormone to be administered with the purpose of it entering the bloodstream to be distributed to all parts of the body. These types of treatment are delivered in different ways, including pills, skin patches, injections (shot into a muscle or under the skin), and vaginal rings. All these methods can contain both hormones, oestrogen and progestin, or just oestrogen.

Topical hormones are used when very little of the hormone must enter the bloodstream. Also, topical hormones can be placed near the area of the body that needs it. Vaginal rings, vaginal creams, and tablets are critical methods for the delivery of topical hormones.

Oestrogen-Progestin Therapy (EPT) can be administered in two ways. Continuous oestrogen-progestin therapy is where a woman takes a dose of oestrogen-progestin therapy daily. This form of delivery is favoured because there is no intermittent bleeding with it. Sequential (cyclical) oestrogen-progestin therapy is where a woman takes different amounts of oestrogen-progestin therapy on specific days. Oestrogen-progestin therapy can also be given monthly. When done this way, an individual is exposed to less oestrogen-progestin therapy, but Cyclical Oestrogen-progestin therapy can produce intermittent bleeding. Oestrogen-progestin therapy (EPT) is given to women who have not had a hysterectomy. The risk of developing endometrial cancer (cancer of the uterus) has been found to occur with oestrogen hormone replacement therapy. The addition of Progestin to therapy has been found to decrease this risk.

The Side Effects of HRT

Some women will not have any side effects from receiving HRT. Like all medications, HRT is also sometimes found to produce adverse side effects. The side effects of HRT are like those experienced by users of oral contraceptives. Some women will not have any side effects from receiving HRT. Potential side effects to look out for include:

- Breakthrough bleeding, vaginal spotting and vaginal yeast infections.
- Painful or tender breasts.

- Skin changes.
- Excess growth of body hair or hair loss.
- Weight gain.
- Mastalgia (breast pain) caused by HRT.
- Headaches and dizziness.
- Stomach cramps, bloating and fluid retention.
- Nausea and vomiting.
- Muscle spasms.
- Neck and throat pain.

HRT and The Risk of Cancer

The two main types of HRT are a combination that contains oestrogen and progesterone or therapy that only includes oestrogen. It has been found that both therapies affect breast cancer risks. According to breastcancer.org, HRT increases the risk of breast cancer by about seventy per cent. It also claims that oestrogen-only HRT increases the risk of breast cancer only if therapy is used for longer than ten years. However, there has been a link to the increase of ovarian cancer due to HRT. The dose of HRT influences breast cancer risk.

When looking at the risks of taking HRT, the common denominator is the length of time that a woman receives HRT, and when she receives HRT. There is an increased likelihood that breast cancer will be found at an advanced stage of development and that the patient will die from breast cancer. There has also been a link found between higher doses of HRT and the risk of breast cancer.

The risk of breast cancer is the same for bioidentical and synthetic hormones. Bioidentical is a hormone replacement that is identical to the hormones the body produces. Bioidenticals are plant-based, so there is some thought that they are more natural compared to synthetic hormones and are chemically the same as the hormones that you find in your body.

If you have been tested for the breast cancer gene and have found out you are at high risk for breast cancer, it is advised that you do not start HRT. A long-term study investigating women with a high risk of breast cancer undergoing HRT has yet to be conducted. However, the medical community is still cautioning women with a high risk, to avoid HRT.

Ovarian cancer has been linked to HRT. It is hard to know how high the risk for ovarian cancer would be since ovarian cancer is rare. A recent analysis of multiple studies concluded that women receiving HRT containing oestrogen and progestin postmenopause did have an increased risk of ovarian cancer. The risk increased for women who were taking the hormones and decreased as they stopped taking HRT.

Although colorectal cancer and lung cancer did not seem to be linked to HRT, there are some findings that women who were taking HRT were more likely to have more advanced cancers such as colorectal cancer. Moreover, HRT was linked to a higher risk of dying from lung cancer. The risk of endometrial cancer is higher among women who took systematic oestrogen therapy (ET). Systematic oestrogen therapy is when a dose is given continuously. This group had a higher risk even after they stopped taking systematic oestrogen therapy. Women who took the pill, patch, or the higher dose vaginal ring were all at high risk for endometrial cancer.

An Analysis of the Studies Done on HRT

In 1991, the National Institute of Health US, led by Dr Bernadine Heally, introduced The Women's Health Initiative. The initiative aimed to analyse the risks and benefits of the treatment of the menopause. It was the most extensive and expensive clinical research ever conducted on women's health. The study was very comprehensive. However, the results of the study were released in a way that was misconstrued by the general public. The press and others concluded that there were high risks attached to the use of HRT. Specifically, there was an increased risk of breast cancer, strokes, thrombosis and heart attacks.

Then, in 2003, The Million Women study published their results. The study concluded that HRT causes breast cancer. Ten years after these studies were undertaken, researchers analysed the findings. The researchers concluded that the original results were limited and that there was more to the study. For example, one of the studies was criticised because they studied women who were ten years post-menopausal, and already had damage to their brain cells. They reported that according to the study, the benefits of HRT outweigh the risks. Overall, the method of analysis and the presentation of facts in these studies were criticised for being unreliable.

Even though some significant studies have deemed HRT safe, there have not been enough long-term studies carried out to determine the actual level of safety regarding the use of HRT. Long-term studies about the health of women receiving HRT still needs to be done. The handling of test results has had a significant impact on the psyche of women around the world. Once a widespread solution to the symptoms of the menopause, HRT is now avoided by many women because of fear. The rush to solve the menopause "problem" with alternative therapies has left some women vulnerable as they try solutions that have not been tested for effectiveness and safety. As science progresses, hopefully, there will be a solution that causes no potential adverse side effects on the body and brain.

Chapter Summary

There are several hormones given to women to help them with the symptoms of the menopause. When a woman is prescribed hormones, it is called Hormone Replacement Therapy (HRT). This type of therapy can control and diminish the overwhelming experience of the menopause. Over the years, the use of HRT has become controversial. There is evidence supporting HRT, but there is also evidence that causes concern. Specifically, HRT in high doses may cause cancer. In the next chapter, you will discover what the alternatives to HRT are.

Chapter Six: What are the Pros and Cons of Using Natural Alternatives to HRT?

Very often, we hear that natural is better. Natural and organic products dominate the grocery store. For example, you can buy premium-priced produce, meats, and dairy. The idea that something is better because it costs more is ingrained into our collective mind. We often know better, but we reach for organic or higher priced alternatives over the generic or sale-priced items. The truth is that the market doesn't always know best. There are quality products that are natural and not overpriced.

If we can't even find the best in the supermarket by price, how can we distinguish care for our menopausal symptoms? There are various menopause remedies available on the market that women have purchased to reduce their symptoms. Many women have chosen to use natural remedies. But do these natural remedies work?

Most of these therapies have been tried by someone we know or even family members. Consequently, they recommend that you buy or use the same thing to relieve your menopausal symptoms. Other natural therapies have been around for a very long time. Does this mean that these remedies have been time-tested by women and have grown popular due to word of mouth?

There are many different therapies available for menopausal women to try for themselves. We will touch on some of these in more depth in chapter seven. Here are some examples of natural remedies that are used by women experiencing the menopause.

Complementary and Alternative (CAM) Therapies

Bioidentical or "natural" hormones are hormone preparations manufactured using hormones that are created from plant oestrogens. These are chemically identical to the hormones our bodies produce. Bioidentical hormones can be taken to replace the hormones in the body that are diminishing with age. Symptoms such as hot flushes, night sweats, mood changes, memory loss, and sleep issues can be helped when you take bioidentical hormones. The bioidentical hormones that are most replicated are oestrogen, progesterone, and testosterone.

There is one key difference between bioidentical hormones and the hormones used in HRT. Bioidentical ones are made from plant oestrogens, while HRT hormones are made from the urine of pregnant horses or other synthetic hormones. There is no evidence that bioidentical hormones are better than the hormones of HRT. More testing must be done.

There are various forms of bioidentical hormones such as pills, patches, creams, gels, and even injections. Some forms of bioidentical hormones are made by drug companies, while there are other types of bioidentical hormones made by pharmacists. The latter type of bioidentical hormones are custom-compounded and not FDA approved. The FDA has approved some bioidentical hormones that have estradiol or progesterone. It is important to talk to your doctor about HRT or taking bioidentical hormones. There are some risks involved so the FDA recommends that if you do have HRT, you take the lowest dose that produces results.

A problem associated with bioidentical hormones and custom-compounded hormones are that they have no regulation. There is no way to vouch for their safety, quality, or purity. It is for this reason that doctors caution their patients about taking these hormones. There have not been enough studies done on these hormones. Consequently, their effectiveness is in question.

Vitamins

If a woman is losing oestrogen during the menopause is, she losing anything else that may cause her to have specific symptoms? Can you relieve a hot flush or night sweat with a vitamin? So far, there is no evidence that vitamins help or cure the symptoms of the menopause. One vitamin that may be helpful is Vitamin D. This vitamin helps to improve calcium absorption, and as we have learned, the loss of oestrogen can make our bones weak.

Traditional Chinese Herbal Medicines

Chinese herbal remedies are popular among many women for taking care of their menopausal symptoms. Ginseng and Dong Quai are two popular herbs that are thought to help a woman during the menopause. Ginseng is a non-toxic adaptogenic plant. Primarily, it can be utilised to help combat the stress encountered by the body. Also, ginseng is believed to increase levels of serotonin and dopamine within the body. This can, therefore, help to improve a person's mood and counteract the negative emotional symptoms associated with the menopause.

While generally safe, ginseng can cause adverse side-effects, including diarrhoea and hypertension. In a systematic review of randomised clinical trials conducted in 2013, it was concluded that the evidence on ginseng as an effective treatment for managing menopause symptoms is limited.

The Dong Quai root is believed to influence estrogen within the body. There has been a limited amount of clinical research conducted on the effectiveness of Dong Quai. One randomised study examined the link between Dong Quai and its effects on hot flushes. The botanical therapy was found to be ineffective in decreasing the rate of hot flushes. However, the study was criticised for not using the same medical formulation of the botanical as used in traditional Chinese medicine. Dong Quai should be used with caution. It cannot be taken by women suffering from different types of blood-clotting conditions or fibroids. As with all herbal medicines, please consult your doctor before taking them.

Soy Products

A popular alternative for relieving the symptoms of the menopause are extracts of the soy plant. Soy extract contains a large concentration of isoflavones. It was believed that this concentration reduced the risk of breast cancer and stopped hot flushes. However, there is evidence that the phytoestrogens in soy extract have a "slight affinity" for oestrogen receptors in women. The issue with soy extracts is that even with the phytoestrogens, it would take a whole lot of soy in your diet to affect your levels.

Red Clover Extract (Promensil)

The red clover (Promensil) is a plant that is thought to be a beneficial and a legitimate alternative to HRT. The plant contains hormone-like chemicals called isoflavones. These chemicals are converted into phytoestrogens by the body. These phytoestrogens are similar to the vital reproductive hormone called estrogen. Therefore, it is believed that red clover extract can help to alleviate the symptoms of the menopause, including hot flushes and breast pain. There have been many studies conducted to study the link between red clover extract and the relief of menopausal symptoms. So far, none of the studies proved that red clover was any better than the placebo given. While the plant is generally safe to use, please be aware it may cause headaches, nausea, vaginal bleeding and muscle aches. Please consult your doctor before using red clover extract.

Black Cohosh (Remifemin)

Black Cohosh is a plant that contains triterpene glycosides. It was used by the Native North Americans to cure fevers and other illnesses. The plant is thought to have curative properties that may relieve symptoms of the menopause. Black cohosh is a plant that contains triterpene glycosides. Glycoside extracts have a weak oestrogenic activity which means that it can act like human oestrogen by binding to a cell's oestrogen receptor location.

Black cohosh has had some success treating menopausal symptoms and has been promoted in lay and medical journals. Specifically, it has become one of the most popular complementary and alternative medicine, or "CAM," for treating menopause symptoms. Black cohosh has an influence, though mild, on hot flushes but there is no evidence it relieves any other symptoms. It has been proven to be better than a placebo for controlling hot flushes. However, the long-term success of black cohosh has been disappointing for some individuals. In tests comparing black cohosh with red clover extract, estradiols and placebos on their effectiveness at helping hot flushes, black cohosh was at the bottom in comparisons. Unlike other natural remedies, black cohosh has been associated with adverse effects.

Evening Primrose Oil

The evening primrose flower contains oils and produces a particular omega fatty acid. Linolenic acid and gamma-linoleic acid is found in the oil of the evening primrose flower. These acids are also found in margarine. It is not harmful, but although it is sometimes recommended to give relief of menopausal symptoms, it has not shown any success in double-blind studies against placebos.

Progesterone Cream

Studies have found that progesterone in a transdermal cream cannot be absorbed in high enough amounts to be effective. Therefore, progesterone cream ought not to be prescribed as a menopause cure.

Wild Yam Cream

Mild yam cream is a desirable choice as an alternative to HRT. It contains diosgenin that can be converted to bioidentical progesterone. Diosgenin alone does not have any effect on menopause symptoms. Wild yam cream cannot be converted outside the laboratory. It is difficult for humans to convert the cream into progesterone.

The Use of Complementary and Alternative Medicine (CAM) Therapies

Since the information that HRT can cause breast and other cancers came to light, women have searched for natural alternatives. These natural alternatives are attractive because, in our society, we believe that anything natural is good. It is said that fifty percent of women have searched for relief by using a CAM. The next level of treatments is over-the-counter-products that flood the market. All of these products sold in stores and advertised as "cures" or relief for menopausal symptoms have not been proven to work better than a placebo. CAMs and over the counter "cures" have not been taken seriously by the medical community, and as a result, there have been no significant studies to promote the efficacy of these products.

Points to consider when looking at natural alternatives:

- Not all-natural alternatives are fully regulated.
- There need to be further studies carried out regarding the effectiveness of natural alternatives.
- Some HRT hormones are made from natural sources, but they have been tested, regulated and researched for safety.

Chapter Summary

There are many alternative treatments for the menopause that are available for women. Alternative medicines are mostly naturally made. These natural medicines are popular among women who are looking for an alternative to synthetic medications. Many alternative medicines have conflicting data about their effectiveness during the menopause. More long-term data and testing of different alternative medicines are needed. In the next chapter, you will discover ways to look after your mental health and wellbeing.

Chapter Seven: How to Look After your Mental Health and Wellbeing During the Menopause

The menopausal journey starts with the onset of the perimenopause and continues through to the postmenopause. This signals the fact that your body has changed and one of the essential hormones in your body is running out. What can a woman do? In the past, many women would take to their beds and wait for their symptoms to go away. Thankfully, the modern woman doesn't miss a beat as she experiences the changes she undergoes during this unique journey. It can be a powerful experience to realise that you will never have a period or ovulate again. Some women get sad that their reproductive years are ending, and some are happy to experience the menopause. Coming to the end of the menopause doesn't mean that this is an end to your life. The journey is just beginning. It is time to take care of yourself better than you ever have before. To do this, you must educate yourself about what is best for your physical and mental health. In this chapter, we will explore the things you need to do for yourself now that you are in the postmenopausal stage of your life.

Therapies to Relax and Calm your Body and Mind

1. **Yoga**

Yoga is a practice that is both spiritual and physical. Various yoga poses stimulate the body and the mind. Yoga uses breathing, exercise, and meditation to spread a feeling of peace both in the mind and body. Practising yoga is a great way to relieve the symptoms of both the perimenopause and the menopause. The balance that you can achieve is very comforting to a body that is going through mental and physical changes. It is also important that you don't overheat your body. However, it is wise to do some exercises that will increase your muscle strength. Here are some poses that are recommended for women who are going through the menopause. Here are some great examples of simple yoga poses that you can try at home. These are the poses that can really make a difference within your body during the menopause:

> ***The Cat - Cow Pose:*** This pose helps to massage your joints and tissues around the spine. The goal is to keep that tissue soft and supple.

> ***The Lunge pose:*** This pose helps you to stretch and free up your breathing so that you can release pent-up tension.

> ***Fan Posture:*** When you get older your muscles begin to shorten and tighten. In particular, your hamstrings and inner thighs shorten. The fan posture is used to stretch these muscles. This pose is also an inversion — meaning that your head is lower than your heart. When this happens, receptors are triggered, and your blood pressure is lowered along with your heart rate and mental activity. This is a very cooling pose.

> ***Sphinx Pose:*** This pose is a suitable alternative to challenging back pain. The sphinx pose is known for its chest-opening posture that stimulates the

sympathetic nervous system. This stimulation both energises and rejuvenates.

***Forward-Facing Hero pose*:** This pose is most important because it stretches the inner thighs and the front of the thighs. It also stretches the spine and is another inversion position that cools the nervous system. This pose also rejuvenates the pelvic region.

2. **Hypnotherapy**

During hypnotherapy, a therapist initiates a trance, and the patient becomes more susceptible to ideas that the therapist is trying to teach the patient. Therapists and patients work together to relieve the mental and physical symptoms of the menopause. Hypnosis can help distract the body from the pain that it is experiencing during the menopause. The calmness achieved with hypnosis can also alleviate feelings of stress and anxiety that tend to surface when your body starts to change. Hypnosis can "dramatically reduce" the frequency of hot flushes and night sweats. In fact, hypnosis may help to relieve hot flushes by as much as eighty per cent. Moreover, hypnosis runs a cool second in reducing the menopause symptoms, just behind hormone replacement therapy. Hypnotic relaxation improves the quality of life and diminishes the experience of anxiety and depression.

In a study conducted at Baylor University in 2012, one hundred and eighty-seven women were observed over a five-week period. The women in the study group had hot flushes that affected their daily lives. In the study, these women were given a weekly session of hypnosis by trained therapists. They were also given audio recordings to use daily. The main visualisations were a snowy path or a cool mountain creek. The results after four weeks showed that the hot flushes diminished by seventy percent. During a three-month follow-up, the decrease in hot flushes averaged eighty percent, while some women reported that they no longer experienced hot flushes at all. During the study, each woman was given skin monitors with electrodes so that when they felt a hot flush coming on, they would push a button and their physiological change, specifically their temperature, was recorded. This gave the study more data on the effectiveness of hypnotherapy, as the monitors recorded the decreasing levels of hot flushes. The outcome of this study was that hypnosis can be safely undertaken by a woman at home to effectively diminish their experiences of hot flushes.

3. **Reflexology**

Reflexology aims to help the body's energy circulate through energy channels and meridians. These techniques are like the ones used in acupuncture and the acupressure of the hands and feet. This kind of therapy can regulate the hormones in the body and can alleviate some of the symptoms of the menopause such as hot flushes and mood swings.

4. **Acupressure**

Acupressure can help relieve the symptoms of the menopause. The principle aim of acupressure is to apply direct pressure upon a network of twelve meridians and balance the flow of positive and negative energy within the body. Ask your doctor if acupressure could work for you. Here is an easy exercise that you can do to help with your menopausal symptoms. Do this exercise for two minutes every other day. Using your thumb, apply pressure to the point that is half a thumb-width above the wrist crease, on the side of your little finger. Apply pressure and firmly circle this point. At the point below the tip of the inside ankle bone, find the acupressure point that is a thumb-width below it. Apply firm pressure using your thumb.

5. **Acupuncture**

Acupuncture is the practice of stimulating certain points on the body with a needle that penetrates the skin to treat various health conditions. Is the practice of stimulating the body to heal itself. Acupuncture has been shown to have a positive effect on menopause symptoms. Symptoms like hot flushes and night sweats can be helped with acupuncture. Acupuncture is a minimal risk procedure but there are some guidelines that you can follow to ensure that you have a positive experience:

- Research information about the clinic that you are going to visit.
- Always visit a licensed practitioner of Acupuncture.
- Begin your session with a discussion of your symptoms and the results you would like to get from your acupuncture session.
- Treatments should only be needed once or twice a week to start and then every two weeks until the symptoms improve.
- Check to see if your health insurance covers acupuncture.

6. **Homeopathy**

Homeopathy can really help with menopause symptoms. The premise behind homeopathy is to consider and treat the body, mind and spirit as a whole. A common medication that is prescribed is Sepia. It is made from cuttlefish ink and can help with the symptoms of depression. Another homeopathic medicine used is Lachesis. Adamas (made from diamond dust) can help with vaginal dryness and reduced elasticity of the vaginal walls due to low oestrogen levels. Another medication that is known to help with weight gain during menopause is Pulsatilla.

7. Aromatherapy and Massage

During an aromatherapy session, a trained aromatherapist uses essential oils to spread certain aromas that will signal well-being to the patient. Aromatherapy can help with stress and anxiety by using specific fragrances to indicate peace and well-being. Touch, in conjunction with therapeutic essential oils, can improve menopausal symptoms. Massage therapy reduces headaches, vanquishes stress and releases endorphins.

There are six main essential oils that are believed to be effective for treating the symptoms of the menopause. These are clary sage, peppermint, lavender, geranium, basil and citrus oils.

Clary sage may be rubbed on the back of your neck or all over your feet. The recommended dose is three drops of diluted sage oil (added to a carrier oil). If you would want a quicker effect, you could add three drops of the diluted sage oil to a tissue and inhale the aroma, exhaling softly. This method will allow the oil to enter your body through your nose. Clary sage helps with symptoms of depression.

Peppermint oil helps with hot flushes and menstrual cramping. Take no more than two drops of peppermint oil. You can administer the peppermint oil by placing two drops on a tissue, breathing in the scent, and exhaling slowly.

Lavender promotes a feeling of relaxation and can help with sleep. Moreover, it is also used to help any perineal pain that you may be feeling. You can relieve a tight or uncomfortable perineum by applying a cold compress with one drop of diluted lavender oil to the area.

Geranium is helpful in relieving stress and anxiety. You can add three drops of the oil to your bathwater or you can add one or two drops to a tissue and inhale the scent. Geranium oil also helps with depression that occurs during the menopause.

Basil can be applied to your feet or the back of your neck to help increase oestrogen levels or to help improve your mood.

Citrus oils help with the overall symptoms of the menopause, and notably, it helps to increase sexual desire. Placing a few drops on a tissue and inhaling the citrus oil is the best way to receive its benefits. Citrus also has anti-inflammatory properties.

Sixty participants took part in a study to determine whether aromatherapy and massage could have an impact on the symptoms of the menopause. Each participant within the experimental group received a thirty-minute aromatherapy session for a total of eight weeks. The participants were treated to a massage with essential oils of lavender, geranium, rose, and jasmine. The aromatherapy massage was given by a certified aromatherapist. The sessions involved abdominal, back and arm massage with essential oils. Each participant enjoyed massages in treatment rooms that had beds warmed by heating pads. The participants who received the massages noticed a reduction of hot flushes, depression, and pain. The researchers believed that the aromatic essential oils had a phytoestrogen effect on the women who received massages with essential oils.

Before using essential oils, consult your doctor to see if this kind of treatment is right for you. It is also wise to consult your doctor, as essential oils may affect any medications that you currently take.

8. **Cognitive Behaviour Therapy (CBT)**

Cognitive Behaviour Therapy (CBT) can help you understand your feelings about the changes occurring inside your body and mind. Cognitive Behaviour Therapy helps with the process of successfully eliminating negative thought patterns. It helps a person to either change their negative thoughts into positive ones or to reduce negative feelings. Cognitive Behaviour Therapy is extremely helpful in dealing with the anxiety and stress that occurs during the menopause.

Here is an example of a practical strategy that a menopausal woman can use to alleviate her stress and anxiety. The main goal of cognitive behaviour therapy in this situation is to create a calmer and more accepting view of the menopause and to respond to stress and anxiety effectively. For example, when you are feeling stressed and anxious, you could write down your reactions and feelings. By writing your thoughts, you have a chance to identify a solid example of what is making you feel anxious or stressed. Once you find the specific thought, you can consider whether the thought is overly negative or threatening. The goal is for you to recognise that your feelings or thoughts can change. For example, you might believe that you cannot handle the stress of your body changing due to the menopause. You often miscalculate your ability to handle the stress.

Further, you often blow the situation out of proportion in your mind. Using cognitive behaviour therapy, you can learn that thoughts are not facts and that they are just one way of viewing what is going on. You can question yourself to find out if there is an actual threat. You could also ask yourself how a calm person would deal with the stress of the menopause or how you would help a friend who was in this situation.

With the success of cognitive behaviour therapy with the menopause, it is plain to see that becoming a person who purposefully changes their thoughts is worthwhile. When you add symptoms such as anxiety and depression into the mix, it is especially important that you pay attention to your thoughts and change what you can.

9. **Paced Breathing**

In order to do this breathing exercise, place your tongue on the roof of your mouth. Breath in through your nose and out through your mouth, pursing your lips. Each time fill your lungs up with air and then release the air completely from your lungs. Count to four when you are inhaling and also when you are exhaling. When you get to the bottom of the exhale, hold your breath for six counts. Try this exercise a maximum of eight times for about two to four minutes in total.

Another breathing exercise is the Anapana respiration, an ancient Buddhist meditation. Breathing and meditating for four to five minutes is the basis of this exercise. While breathing, be very aware of inhaling and exhaling (keeping your mind only on that task). If your mind wanders, go back to concentrating on your breath. Do this for a minimum of five minutes or longer until you feel completely relaxed.

The symptoms the menopause can bring with them a good deal of stress. In fact, stress may be a trigger for some major symptoms like hot flushes. Paced respiration can also be effective in reducing the stress that triggers hot flushes. The ideal situation is for you to take six to eight breaths per minute over a fifteen-minute period. The practice of paced breathing should happen at least twice a day and whenever a hot flush begins. Breathing exercises help to reduce stress and therefore hot flushes as well. Breathing exercises such as slow steady breathing can really help women during the menopause. Practised breathing can do a lot to create a sense of calm. When you are calm, there is less chance that you will trigger the start of a hot flush.

10. Mindfulness

Another effective "mind" strategy is mindfulness. This is the process of focusing your attention on a single moment in the present. Living in the moment can help reduce the symptoms of anxiety. Anxiety is a normal state to experience during the menopause, as a significant change is happening within your body. Try focusing on the present and clear your mind of random thoughts. Whenever you feel anxious, ask yourself what is happening around you in the present moment. The action of being mindful can help you to navigate through the numerous bodily changes of the menopause.

A Mayo Clinic study conducted in 2019, had some positive results with menopausal women who used mindfulness to ease their symptoms. Mindfulness is the act of focusing your attention on the present moment and not passing judgement on your thoughts or sensations. When you are being mindful it is ideal to take a deep breath and observe your space, thoughts and emotions non-judgmentally. Being mindful helped menopausal women deal with negative emotions such as irritability, anxiety, and depression. One thousand seven hundred and seventy women who were menopausal participated in the study. These participants filled out questionnaires and rated their menopausal symptoms, levels of stress and mindfulness. Participants with the highest mindful scores had fewer symptoms of the menopause. These participants scored lower on irritability, depression, and anxiety.

Mindfulness and attitude have a significant impact on your menopause symptoms. It is important to watch your thoughts during the menopause. The absence of positive thoughts can make things much harder to deal with calmly. Try writing in a journal so that you become aware of the thoughts that you are having. At first, try having a small list of positive thoughts to keep in mind. Then expand to more positive thoughts, ever-increasing the amount of positivity in your thinking. In the end, you will find that you have switched your mindset from negative to positive.

The reason mindfulness works so well is that while concentrating on the moment, you can't worry about the future or get sad about the past. Only the present moment matters in your life. Being mindful can feel odd in the beginning. Especially if you are a person who thinks to excess or over-analyses everything. Can you be mindful every minute of every day? Quite frankly, no. However, mindfulness is something you can practice. At first, be mindful for just five minutes and then increase the time in slow increments. Use the mindfulness technique when you feel overwhelmed and ready to explode. Take time to focus on one moment at a time and your mindfulness technique will improve the quality of your life.

Four Simple Mindfulness Techniques

You can practice ***mindful breathing*** either sitting down or standing up. All you must do is breath in and out slowly for a few seconds. Make sure that you are breathing through your nose and exhaling through your mouth. Let your mental checklists and other thoughts just float away. Focus on your breathing until you are completely calm and relaxed.

Mindful observation can help you to focus and clear your mind. Pick a natural item like a rock, a flower, or even a cloud. Focus on that object for two minutes. Relax and focus on this item and look at it like you have never seen it before. Closely examine that object and connect with its energy and the reason for its existence.

Mindful awareness is when you focus on a simple task that you do each day and study it. The point is to stop what you are doing and just be mindful of the task that you are doing. For instance, opening your refrigerator every morning to take out milk or juice. How do you feel at that moment? What is going to happen next? You can also be mindful of a thought that you have every day. Perhaps you think of something negative when you are brushing your teeth. Focus on that thought and how you can change it to be a more positive thought. Then, make it a habit to think of that new and more positive thought from that day forward.

Mindful listening is when you listen to something without preconception. For this exercise, you might want to use headphones. Try to find a radio station or song that you have never heard before. With the headphones on, close your eyes and listen to this new song. Without trying to sort the song into a genre or time period, just listen to the song in a neutral manner. Do not judge. Allow yourself to fall into the music and listen to it differently than before. Listen to every beat and element of the song and get lost in each moment. This is an effective way to relax and get rid of any distressing thoughts.

Mindfulness and being present is a safe way to lower the effects that your menopausal symptoms have on your body and your mind. Let go and live in the moment and believe that some of your symptoms will become less intense and even vanish altogether.

Enter Laughter

Sometimes you can feel like the menopause is not a laughing matter. However, you might find that if you loosen up and allow yourself to see the funny side of life, your attitude will change, and your menopausal symptoms become easier to deal with. You could take a few moments to watch something funny on the internet or perhaps watch a few minutes of your favourite female comic do a routine about the menopause or just being a woman. It can tickle your funny bone enough to make you laugh. Try making laughter a habit. Find the humorous side to hot flushes. It can be done!

Taking Time for Yourself

Life can be very hectic. Situations involving family or work life can exhaust you, so it is important to have a release for your busy and stressful thoughts. The first step is to take control of your schedule and factor in some time for yourself. At first, it might just be a few minutes but as time continues, you will get better at finding moments just for you. Sometimes joining a class or group activity makes it easier to transition from never having time to yourself to set aside one hour a week for a class that gives you some peace of mind. If you take a class to develop a new hobby that is the first chunk of time that you are taking. Then later, you might begin to carve out some time to practice the hobby that you learned in the class. Slowly, you are making time for yourself and before you know it, your stress level is the lowest it has ever been.

Circle of Friends

Things haven't changed so much from the past when the women in your family group were around to give sage advice about going through the menopause. Of course, the menopause has not changed all that much. What has changed is that families are now further apart, and, in some cases, families live in different countries from each other. So where can you get your sage advice? Develop your own circle of friends to help you get through the menopause. Remember high school where there was safety in numbers? The same can be said about the menopause. More minds to solve a problem or a challenge is a good thing.

You might find other like-minded women that also need to form a support group. Women who take part in support groups are better equipped to handle life's changes. When you can talk about your feelings to an empathetic group, you will be better able to put a positive face on something that feels negative in the beginning. If it feels a bit daunting to approach a group of women, start with just one woman at a time. In your life, there are already women who care about you. Just figure out how to gather these women into a support group that can help you get through the menopause.

Emotional Stress and The Menopause

The menopause can be an intensely emotional and stressful time for both yourself and your loved ones. So, you must do things to help you relieve your stress like exercising, setting aside free time, and scheduling fun activities for yourself. Organise your workload and prioritise tasks to ensure you have time for yourself. Be mindful of your day and try not to get overwhelmed. Be in the "now" and avoid worrying about the events in your life. Keep a list of things that bring you peace and carry it around in your purse or wallet so that you can see it, read it, and remember to relax.

Most importantly, don't forget to breathe. Try a common breathing technique called the four-seven-eight for times when you are anxious or in a panic. Slowly and calmly, let all the air out of your lungs and then breathe in through your nose, counting for a total of four seconds. Hold your breath for seven seconds and finally let that breath out for eight seconds. Simply repeat this simple exercise as many times as you need.

Chapter Summary

The menopause can bring about significant changes in a woman's body. These changes can be disruptive. Although Hormone Replacement Therapy (HRT) is readily available, there are treatments other than hormone replacement therapy for the menopause.

Alternative therapies like yoga or acupuncture can help with the changes brought about by the menopause. It is essential to discuss with your doctor what treatments will be best for you. Preparing for your visit to the doctor and preparing questions ahead of time can ensure that you get the answers that you need. The menopause can be overwhelming, but there are things you can do to make it less so. In the next chapter, you will discover how to handle relationships while you are going through the menopause.

Chapter Eight: Maintaining Good Relations at Home and Work

Due to the emotional nature of the menopause, some moods are prompted by our circumstances. It is good to be honest about your feelings with your friends and family so that they can understand how difficult the different mood swings are. If they know what is going on and that your menopause drives your mood, it will be easier for family and friends to handle your behaviour.

Forgetfulness: Being forgetful and living in a sort of brain fog can cause some problems with friends and family. Take notes about important things and celebrations that you need to attend. Do your best not to forget something important. Ask for help from your family and friends.

***Irritability*:** Without knowing that you are doing it, you may be short with your family, co-workers, and friends. You might say things you do not mean because you are not feeling like yourself. Be humble and apologise when you can make amends.

***Weepy*:** You may experience sudden tears or burst into sobs over things that never mattered before. You can cry for no reason, and you feel that your tears are out of control. When this happens, ask for support. Schedule events that make you happy or will cheer you up.

Build your Support Network

Although you may feel out of control with your feelings and emotions, it is crucial that you find support. You don't have to go through the menopause alone. Others can be there to help you on your journey through the menopause. **Here are some suggestions on how to get that vital support:**

***Friends*:** Be open with your friends and ask for their help. Seek out friends who have already gone through the menopause for advice. Schedule "dates" to do fun things that will take your mind off your symptoms. Perhaps lunch with a friend or a movie with your teenagers. A special date-night with your partner or close friend can give you something to look forward to during the week.

***Family*:** Find family members that have gone through the menopause and ask for their advice on how they coped with the menopause. Let your parents or siblings help you with tasks that you find overwhelming (like taking your teenagers for a weekend trip) so that you can have some time to yourself.

***Medical experts*:** Seek out professionals that can help you learn more about the menopause. Go to symposiums or workshops about the menopause.

***Faith-based experts*:** If you are religious, you could look for church support groups or counsellors that can help you cope with the menopause and spiritually.

***Mental health professionals*:** Counsellors, therapists, psychologists, social workers, and psychiatrists can help with the overwhelming feelings that come from mood swings, depression, and anxiety brought about by your menopause symptoms.

Women and the Workplace

Menopausal women are the fastest-growing demographic in the workforce. According to the Faculty of Occupational Medicine (FOM), nearly eight out of ten menopausal women work full-time. Work is good for menopausal women because there is a sense of fulfilment and identity attached to having an occupation. Self-esteem may also be boosted through promotions or the admiration of fellow workers.

Some conditions may exist at work that cannot be altered or controlled by the working woman.

Environments that are temperature controlled can be challenging when a woman experiences hot flushes or night sweats during the day. At home, the menopausal woman can turn down the heating or change into loose clothing. But at work, she must wear work clothes that might not be conducive to comfort. Many women must work in cubicles or small areas with poor ventilation. Also, mood swings and anxiety caused by hormonal fluctuations can cause a woman to feel alienated from her peers if she is working in an enclosed area like a cubical.

Women going through the perimenopause or menopause are in a unique situation. They are not sick, although some symptoms can be debilitating, they do not qualify as a disability excusing them from work or legitimising the need for special accommodations. The topic of the menopause is often taboo. It's difficult for a woman to express any discomfort with her peers. It can be embarrassing even if they are also experiencing the symptoms of the perimenopause and menopause. A modern work environment is diverse, and some people would be offended by open talk of the symptoms of the menopause, for example, talking about the loss of interest in sex.

The competitiveness of the office environment often makes a woman feel like they will be regarded as inferior or the weaker sex if they talk openly about the menopause or ask for any accommodations. The relationship between a menopausal woman and her manager may become strained. A manager may not understand some of the symptoms of the menopause. Emotional upheavals might seem like the woman has a mental illness, and like the menopause, mental illness awareness often falls short of getting sympathy or empathy. The menopause can be easily misunderstood by those unaware of the situation. However, a menopausal woman can work towards making her manager more aware of menopausal symptoms and treatments. Sensitivity training can make a manager or boss predisposed to gain an understanding of the menopause situation.

In the United States, the menopause is not considered a disability by the Americans with The

Disabilities Act. Therefore, an employer does not have to make accommodations for their menopausal employees. However, they may choose to make accommodations such as extra break times for the menopausal employee. It would help the employee to deal with fatigue or mood swings that can benefit from rest and the opportunity to meditate and be mindful.

In the United Kingdom, the Government Equalities Report on the menopause, emphasises the importance of all employers creating training programmes to facilitate a clear understanding of the menopause. The report recommends reasonable modifications like desktop fans or an extra uniform and flexible working. Overall, a manager should foster a work environment that is comfortable both in attitude and awareness. Women who have been through the menopause can support other women in the office who are going through the same experience. Co-workers can be educated informally about the menopause and its accompanying symptoms. This practical step would help to make the menopause less taboo within an office environment.

The Menopause and Family Life

When a family member begins the journey through the perimenopause, there are changes to be made. First, children of any age need to learn sensitivity towards their mother or grandmother. Educating and making children aware that their family member is going through changes that affect her daily life is very reasonable. Daughters need to be told that there is nothing to be afraid of in their future. So often, it does not occur to a mother to ask for special treatment during the menopause. It may be because her children are older and talking about anything with them is difficult. Often, especially in the perimenopause, a woman does not realise that her symptoms are due to the menopause. So, she does not think to ask for special treatment or encouragement from her family.

Tips for explaining the menopause to your children

It is hard for a busy woman to make time for herself. However, she should not be afraid to educate her family about the menopause and the symptoms she is experiencing daily. Here are some points that you can engage your children during a conversation to help increase the menopause-awareness.

K.I.S.S: Keep It Simple Stupid (well, not stupid but you get the point).

Make sure to tell your children that you are okay. Discuss with them that this is a natural process (like losing your teeth or getting taller), that you are not sick, and the symptoms will eventually stop. They need to know that nothing serious is going to happen and that you will not be leaving them. Make the discussion age-appropriate for your child or family members. Your children will not understand some symptoms like sexual dysfunction or breast pain. However, there are some topics like fatigue, hot flushes, and night sweats that can be easily explained to children of any age.

Open a discussion about your mood swings and set ground rules for when you need some time to yourself or a "time-out." Discuss with them a word or phrase that you will use when you are having difficulties and need some time to yourself to get over your negative mood. Let your children know that you are not mad at them and that your aggravation is not directed at them. Give examples about how they could act when you're having mood swings or outbursts. Model for the children the best way to deal with a tough situation. It is okay to tell them that a hormonal imbalance causes your mood swings and that this condition will not last forever.

Make your symptoms relevant to them. Many of the symptoms can be explained to children by giving examples and having a compare and contrast discussion. Symptoms like joint aches and itchy skin can be compared to something they have gone through like chickenpox, measles, or the day after a sports event. Connect with your children and help them to understand that the menopause is not something out of their scope of experience.

Younger children tend to have a limited attention span, so you need to get the relevant points across to them quickly and without any confusion. Tell a story or use visual aids. You could use a doll or stuffed animal to explain how you would like them to treat you when you are having a difficult time with your symptoms. Teenagers love humour, so keep the chat informal and don't be afraid to use fun to lighten up the discussion.

The Menopause and Your Partner

The relationship with your partner is a delicate thing. Between the stages of the perimenopause, the menopause and the postmenopause, many changes have happened to your body. Some of these changes may alienate your partner. Often women suffer in silence and try to make the best of things. Symptoms like hot flushes and night sweats, depression and anxiety, fatigue and joint aches, vaginal dryness and lower libido may put a strain on your marriage. Just as you discussed the menopause with your children, prepare an information "packet" for your partner.

If you can't find time to discuss these changes with your partner, write them an email with a link to a website that will explain the menopause or find a YouTube video that they can watch when they have some downtime. Sometimes family life and work demands make it hard to sit and have the long discussion you want with your partner. Be prepared mentally with topics that you can discuss with them when time allows.

Tell them the difference between the perimenopause and the menopause. Define the menopause for them and tell them about the biological processes that are happening to you. The menopause may start suddenly, the moment when you release the last egg, and the production of oestrogen ceases. However, sometimes the menopause has extended symptoms since you are losing the production of oestrogen from the ovaries. Be open about how you feel now that you can't have children anymore or your feelings about the menopause ushering in a new era for you. Discuss with your partner why sex may be different for you now. If things are very serious, invite your partner to go with you to your health care provider. You can both learn how to have a satisfying sex life, despite some of the symptoms of the menopause.

Make it clear that the menopause will be significant and that it won't be over in just a day. Explain to your partner that your menopause experience will be unique. Your friends may not have any symptoms that are worth mentioning, but that is unique to them. Your symptoms and the severity of them will be unique to you and you only. Then be open about what you are going through and make this information relevant by not minimising or exaggerating the symptoms. Be real and frank about what you are going through. Share the list of symptoms that you are aware of and how you are having or might have them. Engage your partner in a discussion about how the menopause symptoms are significant and affect your quality of life.

Educate your partner about the risks and benefits of Hormone Replacement Therapy. Discuss together whether it is the right choice for you. Be open regarding any discussions held with your doctor and what you have decided about Hormone Replacement Therapy. Explain to your partner that a change in your lifestyle is what the doctor ordered. Healthy eating is something that you can do to help deal with your symptoms. Exercise is also essential, and you will need them to cooperate with you and give you time to exercise.

Give your partner a clear description of how they will know what you are going through by explaining and describing these symptoms. Ask them to be empathetic and kind when you are going through a hot flush or night sweats. You might be acting more annoyed or anxious than usual, and this doesn't have anything to do with them. You are not angry or upset about anything that they've done. You might be depressed or have mood swings, and you will need to have time to yourself when this happens. Choose a phrase or word to signal that you need time to yourself to pull it together after an episode of wild emotions. Explain how the menopause will affect them and that you are aware and concerned about their feelings. Explain to your partner that the menopause or the perimenopause is like going on a journey. It is more than just the symptoms you are experiencing; it is also about the change and growth of getting older.

Chapter Summary

When a woman begins her journey through the menopause, she must communicate openly and honestly with both her boss and her family. It is okay, to be frank with children about the menopause. Further, educating your partner can bring about significant changes in the family. Specifically, when a partner understands what is happening during the menopause, they may be more supportive.

There will always be situations that prove challenging when you have symptoms of the menopause that interfere with your daily life. It would be lovely to escape and go to a five-star hotel on the days that the menopause symptoms are at their worst. Instead, we must work and participate in family life. It's easy to forget that one day, the symptoms of the menopause will not be as severe. You will return to the person you used to be and sort out all the conflicts (real and imagined). In the meantime, excellent communication skills will get you through the hardest days. In the next chapter, you will discover easy and practical ways to stay fit and healthy during the menopause.

Chapter Nine: Staying Fit and Healthy During the Menopause

After you experience the first onset of the perimenopause, you must make sure to treat your body with the utmost respect. It is so essential that your body and mind are cared for with love and kindness. Nutrition, exercise, and mindfulness are three simple habits you can develop to have a significant impact on how you progress through the menopause. In this chapter, we will take a closer look at how a nutritionally balanced diet and plenty of exercise can keep you fighting fit during the menopause and beyond.

The Menopause and Healthy Eating Habits

Your body is going through many physical and emotional changes, and you are experiencing a new stage of your life. It is both challenging and all-encompassing.

Hot flushes and night sweats are making you feel out of control, so you must do something for yourself that is within your control. Nutrition is the thing that matters most because it's how you fuel your body. It is vital that at this stage in life, you are giving your body premium fuel. Many women who go through the menopause gain weight around their abdomen. Hormonal changes, specifically the changing levels of oestrogen in your body, are responsible for this weight gain. Further, your changing metabolism and loss of muscle tone are not doing you any favours.

While experiencing the symptoms of the menopause, you may be tempted to eat emotionally, but this isn't what's best for your body. It might be just what you need to get through a stressful event, but you are not doing yourself any favours by eating cakes, cookies, and pies. It's tempting to buy that gorgeous cupcake to treat yourself, but in the long run, it is going to cause your blood sugar level to spike, and that won't feel good at all. Then not only are you stressed but now you have a sugar hangover. Try to steer off these foods and call a friend or go for a walk when you are feeling agitated or low in spirit.

One of the most common conditions in postmenopausal women is insulin resistance. In order to avoid developing insulin resistance in your body, it is crucial to keep your blood sugar level in check. One of the ways to do this is to eat small meals and to eat frequently, keeping your blood sugar at the optimum level. Another thing you can do to keep your blood level at a healthy point is to eat a diet that is low on carbohydrates. Eating foods rich in protein and low in carbohydrates keeps you feeling full longer, and your blood sugar stays balanced.

Try to eat regular meals every three to four hours as this will keep your blood sugar at a healthy level. Plan your meals and snacks and be aware of what category of food that you are eating so that you can keep your diet balanced. If you ingest too many carbohydrates, your blood sugar will spike but snacking on a protein-rich food like cheese will keep you satiated.

If you do one thing for yourself, let that thing be

drinking lots of water. By the time you are thirsty, you are already dehydrated. Always keep a water bottle (non-plastic) with you and drink one half to two-thirds of your body weight in either ounces or litres. For example, if you weigh one sixty pounds, a little over eleven stones, you should drink half of that amount (80oz. or 2.37 litres). It may sound like a lot of fluid to drink in a day, but it is just ten 8oz cups or 0.237 litres. You can easily fit that amount of water into your day.

Being fatigued due to the menopause is a real thing. No matter how much you rest, you still feel tired. It's entirely understandable that when you are tired, you reach for our good friend caffeine. There is always a caffeinated beverage being promoted wherever you go. However, caffeine isn't your friend. If you drink any caffeinated drinks late in the day, you will have trouble getting to sleep at night. If you don't get enough sleep, you'll feel fatigued. So, it is a vicious circle. Cut down on caffeine, and I promise you, life will get better. Some benefits to quitting caffeine are the following: lowering your blood pressure, better sleep, better mood, reduced anxiety, fewer headaches, healthier teeth, and weight loss.

Besides, think of all the precious time you'll be saving not standing in line to get your latest fix.

Alcohol is fun at a party but not so fun when you get home. Alcohol not only brings on hot flushes and headaches, but it also impairs your judgement. The use of alcohol can cause you to make poor choices, like eating party food that is high in calories and low in nutrients.

How to Plan Your Menopause Diet

Just when you are starting your journey into the menopause, it may seem like your life has gotten even busier than before. It is tempting to grab any food that you can find that's ready and available. At a time when you ought to be sitting down to a relaxing, healthy meal, you find yourself in line for fast food. With a little bit of careful thought, planning and time, you can avoid long lines and have a little peace with your meal. Take a day and make a particular time where you plan your meals. Go online or dust off your recipe books and commit to preparing meals that are delicious and good for you ahead of time. If you search, you can find healthy recipes that take no time at all.

Roasting a chicken with simple seasonings like salt, pepper, and lemon makes a delicious protein source that takes only five minutes to prepare for cooking, for example. You can eat it in various meals over the course of several days. You can also pre-cut fruits and vegetables for quick meals and snacks throughout the week. There are now even healthy alternatives for meals and snacks that are available at your grocery store. Packages of snack-size fruits, vegetables, nuts and seed mixes are becoming popular. A handful of almonds added to any snack can stabilise your hunger until you get home, ready to cook.

By taking the time to prepare the ingredients ahead of time, or buying prepped ingredients from the supermarket, you can have a nutritious meal in the time it takes to wait in line for fast food. Eating foods with nutrients like omega -3 fatty acids can also help you to deal with the nutrient depletions that occur during the menopause. Here is a list of foods that can help your mood and overall health:

Tofu (soy) – a rich source of tryptophan.

Salmon – rich in tryptophan and helps to lower cholesterol and blood pressure and a great source of omega-3 fatty acids.

Nuts and seeds – a healthy handful contains tryptophan, fibre, vitamins, and antioxidants.

Turkey – a source of tryptophan.

Broccoli – impacts oestrogen levels and is full of calcium and fibre.

Berries – reduce inflammation and risk of heart disease.

Whole grains – heart-healthy soluble fibre and a good source of vitamin B to help metabolism.

Dairy products – helps your blood plasma, a good source of tryptophan, good for gut health.

Leafy greens – a good source of calcium, magnesium, potassium, vitamin B, and fibre.

Chicken – a good source of protein that helps build muscle mass and bone.

Green tea – promotes longevity, heart health, reduces the risk of several cancers and inflammation.

Soy – a phytoestrogen that can reduce the menopause symptoms.

Flax – full of omega-3s, phytoestrogens, and vitamin B.

Oatmeal – prevents diabetes, weight gain, and inflammation.

The importance of Building a Healthy Plate of Food

Gone are the days when your metabolism was so high, you could eat anything and not gain weight. Eating well-balanced meals filled with the foods you love is a start to putting premium fuel in your tank. There are so many popular diets, including the Keto diet and the Mediterranean diet. You can choose to follow a specific food plan, or you can improvise and create your unique program. However, the critical thing is that you fill your plate with healthy and nutritious foods.

A diet low in carbohydrates and filled with rich nutrients is ideal. Fruits, vegetables, and lean proteins won't let you down. Find recipes that celebrate fresh produce and lean protein. Some protein-rich foods include beans, fish, and chicken. Healthy fats are also good for you. Avocados are rising in popularity, so add it to your diet by turning it into guacamole, and every dish can be a fiesta. Try avoiding any processed and non-processed foods that are high in salt and sugar.

Eating meals that are low in carbohydrates will also help you maintain a healthy weight. Many women who experience the menopause may also experience insulin resistance due to the high amount of carbs that they consume. Carbohydrates are what your cells love. Carbohydrates get converted into glucose that is meant to be absorbed by your cells. The pancreas secretes glucose that acts like a key for letting the glucose get into the cell. When you have high blood sugar, your pancreas secretes more insulin, and then the cells become less sensitive to it. The insulin and blood sugar remain outside of the cell. It prompts the pancreas to think that you need even more insulin, so it secretes more. Eventually, the pancreas is going to shut down from overwork, and you will find yourself becoming a diabetic.

Your parents always said, eat your fruits and

vegetables, and they were right. All fruits and vegetables are very rich in vitamins, minerals, fibre, and antioxidants. Fruits and vegetables are so good for you, filling half your plate with them makes up what many nutritionists like to call a healthy plate. There are many benefits to eating the vitamins and minerals offered by fruit. Prepare containers of fruit and vegetables as your go-to snack. Watch out for fruits like bananas and oranges as they are high in natural sugars.

A woman going through the menopause needs to eat more protein. The U.S. Recommended Dietary Allowance (RDA) for protein is 0.36 grams per pound (9.8 grams per kg) of body weight. Foods high in protein are eggs, meat, fish, legumes and dairy products. Based on the Reference Nutrient Intakes (RNI), a person should have 0.75g of protein for each kilogram that you weigh. For example, if you weigh roughly 11 stone, you should eat about 52.5g of protein a day.

Popular meal plans suggest that you take whole grains out of your diet and stick to proteins and fat. However, there are many benefits to whole grains as they are high in nutrients, fibre, and B vitamins. The National

Institute of Health reports that whole grain cereals are beneficial as they contain phytochemical compounds and are highly nutritious. The consumption of these whole-grain cereals and bread prevents chronic diseases. As with most things, eating whole grains in moderation is recommended.

In the past, you wouldn't see the words "healthy" and "fat" together since there was a campaign to abolish fat in your diet. Today, we possess a great deal more knowledge about fat and its role in our digestion. There is such a thing as healthy fats. Foods such as fatty fishes, including salmon and mackerel, contain high levels of omega-3 fatty acids and should be included in your diet. Seeds like flax, chia, and hemp are also high in omega-3 fatty acids. A diet rich in these foods is essential in protecting your heart. There have also been some studies that support the fact that omega-3s help to reduce hot flushes.

Phytoestrogens are compounds in food that provide a minimum amount of oestrogen in your body. It is controversial because researchers are still trying to figure out how the body processes these types of foods, and if they provide enough oestrogen to make a difference. Foods that have phytoestrogens are soybeans, chickpeas, peanuts, flax seeds (in small amounts), grapes, berries, plums, and green and black tea.

The Menopause and Weight Gain

One of the significant symptoms of the menopause is weight gain. Remember when you were younger, and you made the transition from a teenager to a young adult? Then you could eat anything that you wanted and not put on extra weight. Now your body is changing, and your metabolism is not what it used to be. You no longer burn energy as quickly as when you were younger. Now that you are going through the menopause, you will notice that you are a little bit heavier. The menopause is affecting your metabolism, and you will gain more weight around your abdomen. For some women, it will only be a small weight gain; for others, it will be a more significant, noticeable gain. The menopause is a time when we try to understand the changes that are happening in our bodies. Proper nutrition can help with some of the symptoms of the menopause. Is it a bad thing when we turn to food for comfort? If the foods that you are reaching for are not suitable for you, then this should give you pause. Maybe this is the push you need to change your current eating plans and introduce healthier foods into your diet.

You may have also noticed that your efforts to lose this weight are not as effective as they once were. Do not stress about this. Even though losing weight might be a little more complicated, there are things you can do to bring about weight loss. If you feel that you are overworking yourself, remember that it is perfectly all right to rest or change exercises. It is also not necessary to excessively exercise or starve yourself so that you can lose weight. Treat your body with kindness and care.

The first step you can take is to increase your activity levels slowly. Does your vision of the menopause include sitting on your couch and knitting baby booties for your future grandchildren, or does it involve jumping out of aeroplanes? Find something in the middle and stick to it. Walking for as little as ten minutes a day can boost your metabolism.

Exercise and the Menopause

It seems like there isn't a day that goes by without hearing that exercise is good for us. Some exercise regularly, but in a time where we are fatigued and maybe even a bit unnerved by the symptoms of the menopause, it can be tough to go out and exercise. Some women find opportunities to walk or take an exercise class, and they seem better for it. If exercise is good for you in general, can it also be good for you during the menopause? Is there anything to gain by taking the time to exercise?

The answer is in a study of the menopause conducted in 2011, called *"Exercise beyond the menopause: Dos and Don'ts."* There is no doubt that as you travel through the unique experience of the menopause, you will find it necessary to change your lifestyle. One of the things you can change is to become more active. In this study, researchers found that two hours and thirty minutes of moderate activity each week made an impact on women's health and menopause symptoms.

They found six benefits to exercising:

1. Exercise reduces the metabolic risks associated with declining oestrogen.
2. Exercise burns calories and helps fight against the weight gain experienced during the menopause.
3. Exercise increases bone mass.
4. Exercise reduces low back pain.
5. Exercise reduces stress and improves your mood.
6. Exercise reduces hot flushes.

Even if exercise has not been part of your daily routine, you can start slow and work up to more vigorous activities. Instead of a dull exercise routine, you can do things you enjoy, like walking, cycling, gardening, swimming, or going to an exercise class. Any activity that gets the heart pumping is good. Finding out the exact number of heartbeats you should have per minute is easy with this simple equation. Determine the maximum heart rate for your exercise using the following formula:

220 - (your age) = maximum heart rate (bpm)

So, for example, if I am 34 years old, my formula will look like this: 220 − 34 = 186 (bpm). Therefore, in this example, 186 is the average maximum number of times your heart should beat per minute during exercise.

A good sign that you are exercising at a productive level is to be able to do your exercise without becoming out of breath. A simple guideline to determine whether you are exercising at the right level is whether you can talk and exercise. For example, can you talk when you are walking and not getting breathless? Or, can you say a few words to a friend when you are taking part in aerobic exercise? If you can carry on a conversation, the exercise level is too easy for you.

The study used various exercise methods and suggested weight-bearing, high impact exercises like dancing, high impact aerobics, running or jogging, and stair climbing. If possible, try participating in a group sport like tennis, basketball, or volleyball to add some fun into your exercise routine. The weight-bearing low-impact exercise was also recommended: walking, elliptical training machines, stair-step machines, low impact aerobics, and other group exercise programs like Zumba. Check out your local sports centre or community hall to see what classes are available.

Another area of recommendation was weight and strength training. Some examples were lifting weights, using resistance bands, or weight machines for exercise. The study even recommended some important exercises: squats, shoulder presses, lateral pulldowns, leg presses, seated rows, and the movements practised in Tai Chi. Non-weight-bearing low-impact activities included: cycling, swimming, stretching, and flexibility exercises. Non-impact exercises like Tai Chi were recommended to help with mental focus and calm. Overall the study recommended endurance exercises (aerobic) strength exercise and balance exercises. The researchers felt that a practical exercise prescription was resistance and weight-bearing training three days a week. On the remaining days of the week, brisk walking, cycling, using the treadmill, gardening, or dancing. The researchers also cautioned warming up before starting any exercise.

The study went further to outline the steps menopausal women could take to incorporate exercise into their life.

> ***Step 1***: stretch, walk on a treadmill or go for a brisk walk.
>
> ***Step 2***: take part in an aerobic activity that gets the heart going and burns fat.
>
> ***Step 3***: Lift weights, use resistance bands to keep bones strong.
>
> ***Step 4:*** Become more flexible and practice yoga or Pilates for better muscle function (this also helps reduce anxiety).
>
> ***Step 5***: Remember to cool down at the end of the workout by walking and stretching for a few minutes.

The Conclusions of the Study

The main conclusions of the study included that women can enjoy an increased quality of life even if they do not take HRT, postmenopausal women who exercise benefit by maintaining a healthy body, better bone density levels, and good mental health, that osteoporosis is kept under control with exercise and that moderate levels of training help you maintain a healthy weight, improves muscle mass, strength, balance, and coordination. The conclusions of the study were similar to other findings regarding the benefits of exercise during the menopause. Good things happen to your body when you exercise. It can also be easy to feel isolated during the menopause, so going out to exercise, whether you walk around the block or join an exercise group can also help your mental health.

Chapter Summary

Exercise can help you cope with the symptoms of the menopause. A healthy diet is also an excellent way to counteract weight gain and mood swings that happen during the menopause. Overall, a healthy lifestyle can go a long way to help you deal with the menopause positively and effectively.

FINAL WORDS

In my lifetime I have seen two women go through the menopause; my grandmother and my mother. They never discussed their situations because when my grandmother experienced it, I was in nursery school. Then, when my mother experienced it, I was a teenager. I had more important things on my mind at those times, like nap time and boys. Both women went through the menopause silently and without drama. There were hushed whispers and crying, but I didn't understand the reason.

Now that I am going through my own season of change, I think of my grandmother and my mother, and their solitude. I am so grateful that I don't have to be silent. I am happy that now there are support groups, therapists, and counsellors for when it all gets to be too much. the menopause is no longer a secret that one must suffer in silence over.

In the past, the menopause was the stuff of drama, but the players said their lines in whispers away from polite society. It was a time when mothers sat alone and thought of children they were never going to have. Working women second-guessed their decision to have careers instead of children. And men stayed confused about women's issues.

Today there are doctors and mental health professionals that specialise in treating menopausal women. Although there still are some medical throwbacks who don't take women seriously; most providers listen to their female patients and try to give the best medical relief that they can.

This book is not just about giving information; it is about giving answers. The purpose of this book has been to unravel the mysteries of a woman's transition from menstruation to the menopause. I hope that you have felt my compassion and that I gave to you clear, practical information that was accessible to you in every way.

The state of the menopause comes finally after a period of perimenopausal symptoms. This is a time where your body says: look at me now. See what I need; give me your attention. For some women the menopause passes with barely any recognition and for others, life will never be the same.

I have been honoured to be a small part of your journey. We started this book talking about the beginning of the premenopausal stage of your unique journey. This is the stage that takes us by storm and wakes us up to what is coming for us. There are psychological and physiological symptoms that beg not to be ignored.

This is a confusing time with periods stopping for months and then starting back up again. The symptoms of the perimenopause are like the opening act of a Vegas show – not the real thing but someone who gets us ready for what is to come. In the end, the symptoms of the perimenopause got us to see our doctors because we needed a translation of what we experienced.

Then the menopause came along and the stage was hushed. What does it mean to feel hotter than the sun and to no longer have our monthly periods? How can something we've been dealing with since we were young girls just stop? Even though we went through the perimenopause, we feel taken aback when the menopause starts.

Then there are the psychological effects of the menopause. It is a time of confusion. Our brains are foggy, and we often find ourselves crying for no reason. Then, at the drop of a hat, we are aggravated and annoyed. All our emotions make themselves known all at the same time. We feel crazy and told we are not. It's hard to believe that this is all due to our periods stopping.

But there is more than the cessation of menstruation. It's about our body losing hormones that we have come to depend on: oestrogen, progesterone, and to a certain degree, testosterone. We are shocked at the fact that the hormones we never knew were there had left our bodies with the consequences of symptoms that we never thought would happen to us. Breast pain, thinning hair, aching joints, heart palpitations, itchy skin – some or of all these came to visit and was welcomed like a second cousin, twice removed.

The most important part of this book was to present you with information that empowered you to make the tough decisions about the amount of intervention you wanted for the menopause. There are compelling sides for Hormone Replacement Therapy, natural alternatives or very little intervention at all. This is your journey and your decisions are for you alone. Yet, you are very much not alone.

Your journey through the menopause does not have to be a lonely one. It is important to let our families into our confidence and guide them to what they can do for you during this time. It is wonderful to be out in the open and to be able to embrace the support of our partners, children, extended families and working families.

Remember to treat yourself like you would an important guest in your home. Choose the best foods and eat wisely. Now is not the time to eat in a hurry and grab whatever is available. Plan ahead and make good choices.

Find the time for yourself to exercise not only your mind but also your body. All the things that must get done can wait. Focus on completing the things you need to do for yourself. If exercise is not a priority yet, I challenge you to re-evaluate how important exercise is for you.

Be kind to yourself and ask for help when you need it. Seek out the advice of a mental health professional if the symptoms of the menopause interfere with your daily life. There is no blame or dishonour for reaching out for help with our thoughts and emotions. Lastly, remember that for each symptom of the menopause, there is something actionable that you can do. Whether it is eating certain foods or adding supplements to your life, you can and will take care of yourself. I wish for you the best possible journey through the menopause.

Bibliography

Acupressure Points and Massage Treatment. (n.d.). Retrieved September 11, 2019, from https://www.webmd.com.

Blocker, w. (n.d.). perimenopause Early Symptoms, Signs, Age, Test, Remedies & Treatments. Retrieved September 9, 2019, from http

British Homeopathic Association. (n.d.). Retrieved September 11, 2019, from https://www.britishhomeopathic.org/charity/how-we-can-help/articles/womens-health/menopausal-symptoms/

Chang, L. (2005, July 18). Your Brain on the menopause. Retrieved September 9, 2019, from https://www.webmd.com/the menopause/features/your-brain-on-the menopause.

Changes in Hormone Levels, Sexual Side Effects of the menopause | The North American the menopause Society, NAMS. (n.d.). Retrieved September 9, 2019, from https://www.the menopause.org/for-women/sexual-health-the menopause-online/changes-at-midlife/changes-in-hormone-levels

Cherney, c. (2019, March 8). Prethe menopause, perimenopause, and the menopause. Retrieved

September 9, 2019, from https://www.healthline.com/health/the menopause/difference-perimenopause

Clinical hypnosis can reduce hot flashes after menopause. (n.d.). Retrieved September 11, 2019, from https://www.sciencedaily.com/releases/2012/10/121024111526.htm

Cognitive Behaviour Therapy (CBT) for Menopausal Symptoms. (2018, August 7). Retrieved from https://www.womens-health-concern.org/help-and-advice/factsheets/cognitive-behaviour-therapy-cbt-menopausal-symptoms/.

Dresden, D. (2017, May 22). What causes mood swings during the menopause? Retrieved September 9, 2019, from https://www.medicalnewstoday.com/articles/317566.php

Effective Treatments for Sexual Problems, Sexual Side Effects of the menopause | The North American the menopause Society, NAMS. (2019). Retrieved September 9, 2019, from https://www.themenopause.org/for-women/sexual-health-the menopause-online/effective-treatments-for-sexual-problems

Evans, J. R. (2018, April 27). Bioidentical Hormone Replacement Therapy. Retrieved from https://www.healthline.com/health/bioidentical-hormone-replacement-therapy.

Expert Answers to Frequently Asked Questions About Menopause. (n.d.). Retrieved from https://www.menopause.org/for-women/expert-answers-to-frequently-asked-questions-about-menopause

FDA Office Of Women's Health. (2017). *the menopause and Medicines to Help You*. Retrieved from https://www.fda.gov/media/119387/download

Gary R. Elkins, William I. Fisher, Aimee K. Johnson, Janet S. Carpenter, Timothy Z. Keith. Clinical hypnosis in the treatment of postmenopausal hot flashes. the menopause: The Journal of The North American the menopause Society, 2012; DOI: 10.1097/gme.0b013e31826ce3ed

Ginseng for menopause sleep problems | Healthspan. (n.d.). Retrieved September 11, 2019, from https://www.healthspan.co.uk/advice/get-into-ginseng-how-to-get-to-sleep-during-menopause

Gotter, A. (2018, May 7). Low Progesterone: Complications, Causes, and More. Retrieved September 9, 2019, from https://www.healthline.com/health/womens-health/low-progesterone

Herbal Remedies for Menopause, Menopause

Information & Articles | The North American Menopause Society, NAMS. (n.d.). Retrieved September 11, 2019, from https://www.menopause.org/for-women/menopauseflashes/menopause-symptoms-and-treatments/natural-remedies-for-hot-flashes.

How much protein is it safe to eat? - BBC Food. (2019, August 27). Retrieved from https://www.bbc.co.uk/food/articles/should_you_worry_about_how_much_protein_you_eat.

How to Manage Your menopause Symptoms with Acupressure Therapy? (n.d.). Retrieved from https://medicaladvice.knoji.com/how-to-manage-your-the menopause-symptoms-with-acupressure-therapy/.

How Will I Know I'm in the menopause? the menopause Stages, Symptoms, & Signs | The North American the menopause Society, NAMS. (n.d.). Retrieved September 9, 2019, from https://www.the menopause.org/for-women/the menopauseflashes/the menopause-symptoms-and-treatments/are-we-there-yet-navigate-now-with-our-guided-the menopause-tour

HRT and alternatives. (2019). Retrieved September 9, 2019, from https://www.rcog.org.uk/en/patients/the menopause/hrt-and-alternatives/

https://www.health.harvard.edu/womens-health/perimenopause-rocky-road-to-the menopause. (n.d.). Retrieved from https://www.health.harvard.edu/womens-health/perimenopause-rocky-road-to-the menopause

Hur, M. H., Yang, Y. S., & Lee, M. S. (2008). Aromatherapy massage affects menopausal symptoms in Korean climacteric women: a pilot-controlled clinical trial. Evidence-based complementary and alternative medicine: eCAM, 5(3), 325–328. doi:10.1093/ecam/nem027

Iftikhar, N. (2018, June 20). Treating the menopause with Antidepressants. Retrieved September 9, 2019, from https://www.healthline.com/health/antidepressants-for-menop

Is the menopause Causing Your Mood Swings, Depression or Anxiety? (2015, June 3). Retrieved September 9, 2019, from https://health.clevelandclinic.org/is-the menopause-causing-your-mood-swings-depression-or

Jones, M. (2006). the menopause For Dummies, 2nd Edition. John Wiley & Sons.

Kim, M. S., Lim, H. J., Yang, H. J., Lee, M. S., Shin, B. C., & Ernst, E. (2013). Ginseng for managing menopause symptoms: a systematic review of randomized clinical trials. Journal of ginseng research, 37(1), 30–36. doi:10.5142/jgr.2013.37.30

Menopause. (2019, August 6). Retrieved September 11,

2019, from https://www.nhs.uk/conditions/menopause/

Mindfulness may ease menopausal symptoms. (n.d.). Retrieved September 11, 2019, from https://www.sciencedaily.com/releases/2019/01/190117090449.htm

Mishra, N., Mishra, V. N., & Devanshi (2011). Exercise beyond the menopause: Dos and Don'ts. Journal of mid-life health, 2(2), 51–56. doi:10.4103/0976-7800.92524

Parker Gordon, J. (2016, October 13). Can Essential Oils Provide the menopause Relief? Retrieved from https://www.healthline.com/health/the menopause/essential-oils-for-the menopause.

Patz, A. (2015, December 16). 6 Ways Your Brain Transforms During the menopause. Retrieved from https://www.prevention.com/health/a20491629/the menopause-brain-effects/

Perimenopause: Rocky road to the menopause - Harvard Health. (2009, August 24). Retrieved September 9, 2019, from https://www.health.harvard.edu/womens-health/perimenopause-rocky-road-to-the menopause

Principles of homeopathy. (2003). *Homeopathy*, 92(4), p.232.

Rabbitt, M. (2019, June 10). 3 Simple Breathing Exercises That Ease Hot Flashes. Retrieved from https://www.prevention.com/health/g20486844/breathing-exercises-to-ease-hot-flashes/.

RED CLOVER. (n.d.). Retrieved from https://www.webmd.com/vitamins/ai/ingredientmono-308/red-clover.

Royal College of Nursing. (2017). the menopause RCN Guidance for nurses, Midwives, Health Visitors. Retrieved from file:///C:/Users/jazba/Downloads/PUB-006329%20(7).pdf

Sexual pleasure during and after the menopause. (2017, July 25). Retrieved September 9, 2019, from http://www.fpa.org.uk/sexual-pleasure-during-and-after-the menopause

Silver, N. (2017, April 27). What Health Changes Should You Expect postmenopause? Retrieved September 9, 2019, from https://www.healthline.com/health/the menopause/postmenopausal-health

Speakman, l. (2019, June 12). Your Body On A Hot Flash. Retrieved September 9, 2019, from https://www.prevention.com/health/a20484262/your-body-on-a-hot-flash/

Stöppler, M. (n.d.). the menopause: 10 Questions To

Ask Your Doctor. Retrieved September 9, 2019, from https://www.medicinenet.com/the menopause_10_questions

Taylor, S., Sandy, II, J. B., II, J. B., Fledgerson, B., Fledgerson, B., … Meditation Claremont. (2017, October 27). 6 Mindfulness Exercises You Can Try Today. Retrieved from https://www.pocketmindfulness.com/6-mindfulness-exercises-you-can-try-today/.

The menopause & Depression, Mood Changes | The North American the menopause Society, NAMS. (2019). Retrieved September 9, 2019, from https://www.the menopause.org/for-women/the menopauseflashes/mental-health-at-the menopause/depression-the menopause

The menopause and Hormones | National Center for Health Research. (2018, June 14). Retrieved September 9, 2019, from http://www.center4research.org/the menopause-and-hormones/

The menopause and work: why it's so important. (2019, March 10). Retrieved September 9, 2019, from https://the menopauseintheworkplace.co.uk/the menopause-at-work/the menopause-and-work-its-important/

The menopause Mood Swings | Hormone Health Network. (n.d.). Retrieved September 9, 2019, from https://www.hormone.org/diseases-and-conditions/the menopause/the menopause-mood-swings

Tworek, T. (2018, December 13). Symptoms of the menopause and Treatment Options. Retrieved September 9, 2019, from https://www.bodylogicmd.com/for-women/the menopause-symptoms

Using HRT (Hormone Replacement Therapy). (2017, November 10). Retrieved September 11, 2019, from https://www.breastcancer.org/risk/factors/hrt

Villines, Z. (2018, July 16). How does perimenopause affect periods? Retrieved September 9, 2019, from https://www.medicalnewstoday.com/articles/322480.php

Waston, K. (n.d.). Acupuncture and the menopause. Retrieved December 18, 2017, from.

Weber, M. T., Rubin, L. H., & Maki, P. M. (2013, May). Cognition in perimenopause: the effect of transition stage. Retrieved from https://www.ncbi.nlm.nih.gov/pubmed/23615642.

WebMD - Better information. Better health. (n.d.). Retrieved September 11, 2019, from https://www.webmd.com/vitamins/ai/ingredientmono-936/dong-quai.

What questions should I ask my doctor about the menopause? | the menopause. (n.d.). Retrieved September 9, 2019, from [https://www.sharecare.com/health/the menopause/what-question-ask-doctor-](https://www.sharecare.com/health/the-menopause/what-question-ask-doctor-)the menopause

Wicks, L., & Wicks, L. (2019, April 8). The 12 Best Foods to Eat During the menopause. Retrieved from https://www.cookinglight.com/nutrition-101/best-foods-for-the menopause-diet.

Wiley, T. S., Taguchi, J., & Formby, B. (2004). *Sex, lies, and the menopause: the shocking truth about synthetic hormones and the benefits of natural alternatives*. New York, NY: Perennial Currents.

Wren, B. G. (2013). *The Menopause: Change, Choice and HRT*. Summer Hill, N.S.W.: Rockpool Publishing.

Zinman, R. (2017, April 19). 5 Gentle Yoga Poses for the menopause. Retrieved from 5 Gentle Yoga Poses for the menopause#1.

Milton Keynes UK
Ingram Content Group UK Ltd.
UKHW041306140124
436019UK00003B/62

9 781692 339692